THE VAGUS NERVE

DAVE FR HUNTHER

Copyright © 2019 by Dave FR Hunther

The aim of this piece is to provide accurate and reliable information on the topic and issue covered. The publication is marketed with the assumption that no accounting, legally licensed or otherwise eligible resources are provided by the publisher. A specialist in the field should be requested if advice is appropriate, legal, or professional.

From a Declaration of Principles that a Commission of the American Bar Association and a Committee of Publishers and Associations embraced and approved fairly.

The copying, duplication or dissemination of any portion of this text in either digital or written format is in no way legal. Recording of this publication is totally prohibited, and it is not permissible to archive this paper unless the publisher gives written permission. Reserved for all rights.

The information provided herein is claimed to be accurate and reliable, since any fault, in terms of inattention or otherwise, resulting from any use or misuse of any procedures, processes or instructions found therein is the full and absolute responsibility of the receiver user.

Under no conditions will any civil responsibility or blame be taken against the publisher, whether directly or indirectly, for any restoration, harm or financial loss due to the details found herein.

The copyrights not kept by the publisher are owned by corresponding authors.

The information contained herein is solely and universally available for information purposes. The information is presented without a warranty or promise of any kind.

The trademarks used are without approval, and the patent is issued without the trademark owner's permission or protection. The logos and labels in this book are the property of the owners themselves and are not associated with this report.

TABLE OF CONTENTS

Introduction 1

What Vagus Nerve Is...2

    Cranial Piece Of The Vagus Nerve 3

    Cervical Piece Of The Vagus Nerve................................4

    Thoracic Piece Of The Vagus Nerve...............................8

    The Abdominal Portion Of The Vagus Nerve...............8

    Left Vagus Nerve 12

    Right Vagus Nerve 13

The Sympathetic And Parasympathetic Nervous System ...15

    Branches 17

    Innervation..18

    The Vagus Nerve And The Heart..................................20

    The Capacity Of Vagus Nerve.......................................21

    Vn As Modulator Of Intestinal Immune Homeostasis 30

Functions Of Vagus Nerve 35

    The Vagus Nerve Prevents Inflammation. 35

    It Helps You Take Memories. 36

    It Helps You Breathe. 36

    It's Intimately Involved With Your Heart....................36

    It Initiates Your Body's Relaxation Response. 37

    It Translates Between The Gut And Brain. 37

    Over-Stimulation Of The Vagus Nerve Is The Most
    Common Cause Of Fainting..37

    The Electrical Stimulation Of The Vagus Nerve
    Diminishes Inflammation And May Inhibit It
    Altogether. 38

- Vagus Nerve Stimulation Has Developed A New Field Of Medicine. 38
- Vagus Nerve Testing 39
  - Vagus Nerve Issues 39
- The Potential Effects Of Vagus Nerve Dysfunction 41
- Signs And Symptoms Of Vagus Nerve Dysfunction 42
- Vagus Nerve Disorder 44
- Vagus Nerve Stimulation (Vns) 64
  - Gadget And Method 64
  - Vns Therapy 65
  - The Neural Mechanism Of Vns 70
- Yoga 75
  - When Exposed To Cold 82
  - Breathing 83
  - Effects On Mental And Physical Health 84
- Vagus Nerve Stimulation (Continued) 85
  - Benefits Of Vagus Nerve Stimulation 85
  - Add Fish To The Eating Regimen 85
  - Become A Yogi 85
  - Form Social Associations 86
  - Generously Chew Gum 86
  - Hack Or Agreement The Stomach Muscles 86
  - Eat More Fiber 86
  - Engage The Larynx 86
  - Exercise Routinely 87
  - Fast Irregularly 87
  - Discover An Acupuncturist 87

Get Immediate Daylight 87
Incorporate Petition Each Day 87
Giggle Regularly 88
Figure Out How To Adore Cold Temperatures 88
Think Every Day 88
Practice Tai Chi 88
Have Kneaded Regularly 89
Rest On The Correct Side 89
Invest Some Energy With Nervana 89
Supplement Zinc And Serotonin (5-Htp) 89
Attempt A Douche 90
Utilize Pulsed Electromagnetic Field (Pemf) Treatment 90
Work The Vocal Harmonies 90
A Germaine Note On Gluten And The Vagus Nerve .. 90
Past Without Gluten Foods 91
Against Neuroinflammation Or Immunomodulation .. 92
Methods Of Action Of Vns For Epilepsy 94
Instruments Of Activity Of Vns For Comorbidities Related To Epilepsy 96
Neuropsychiatry 97
Adenosine And Epilepsy 98
Adenosine And Comprehension 98
Adenosine And Also Depression 99
Aetna 100
Vagus Nerve Obstructing For Being Obese. 102
Vgn For Better Digestion 115

Role Of Vagal & Spinal Sensory Pathways On Ecc's Activity 119
Vagus Nerve As Modulator Of Brain-Gut Axis 121
   The Vagus Nerve Manipulates Your Hunger Level 123
Anatomy Of The Vagus Nerve 128
   Definition Of The Anatomy Of The Vagus Nerve.... 129
   Vagus-Related Treatment Of Depression 134
   Vagus-Related Treatment Of Psd 140
   Nerve Stimulation For Epilepsy 151
How To Hack Your Vagus Nerve 155
   How Is The Vagus "Hacking" Working? 157
   Food For Your Vagus Nerve And Gut Health 160
   Is The Heart Palpitations And Stomach Bloating Connected? 162
Vagus Nerve Damage Symptoms 166
   What Is The Nervous Illness Of The Vagus? 166
      Muscle Cramps 168
      Fainting 168
      Peptic Ulcer 169
   Treating Vagus Nerve Problems 169
   Reflex Syncope 171
      Signs And Symptoms 172
      Changes In Lifestyle 175
The Vagus Nerve In Trauma Recovery 179
   Trauma And The Vagus Nerve 181
   The Vagus Nerve And Trauma Recovery 182
Conclusion 186

INTRODUCTION

Vagus nerve, also known as the X cranial nerve, also reffered to as the 10th cranial nerve, the cranial nerve's longest and perhaps most complex.

The nerve of the vagus passes from the chest to the abdomen through the head and thorax. It is a combined nerve comprising of fibers for parasympathy.

This piece gives full details about the vagus nerve, its stimulation, its problems, and so much more. Read till the end.

WHAT VAGUS NERVE IS.

The Vagus nerve is the basically longest of the 12 sets of cranial nerves that radiate from the mind. The vagus nerve is definitely the 10th cranial nerve. Just as the glossopharyngeal nerve, it is the most mind-boggling nerve having four cores and five unique sorts of fibers in it.

The vagus nerve is exceptionally all around situated to interface the safe and focal sensory systems.

Since it innervates the organs that are gateways of section or channels for pathogens and their items, it transmits data to or from the outside of the mind to tissues and organs somewhere else in the body.

The name "vagus" originates from the Latin expression for "wandering." This is because the vagus nerve meanders from the cerebrum into organs in the neck, chest, and guts.

Furthermore, it manages a tremendous scope of significant capacities, conveying engine, and physical driving forces to each organ in your body.

There are numerous sensory system capacities gave by the vagus nerve and its related parts.

The vagus nerve is blended, it contains substantial and instinctive afferent fibers, just as general and uncommon instinctive efferent fibers. The vagus nerve fibers start from three cores:

- The nucleus ambiguus,

- dorsal nucleus of the vagus nerve,
- solitary tract nucleus

The nucleus ambiguus consists of assemblies of engine neurons offering an increase into exceptionally instinctive and effective fibers, giving innervation to branchial curved skeletal muscles, for example, cricothyroid tissue, pharynx muscles, and natural larynx muscles.

The vagus nerve's dorsal nucleus has typically instinctual efferent impulses, granting the viscera a parasympathetic innervation.

The distinct tract nucleus (also known as the nucleus of just the single tract) contains neurons that obtain data from unique instinctive afferent fibers that convey objective (right) data of epiglottis, and general afferent instinctual fibers that transmit accurate mucosal data from the delicate feeling of taste, pharynx, and larynx.

The vagus nerve can be partitioned into cranial, cervical, thoracic, and stomach parts.

Cranial piece of the vagus nerve

Rootlets that emerge from the medulla oblongata structure a littler second rate and ale predominant packs that aggregately structure the vagus nerve after it leaves the medulla through the posterolateral sulcus alongside the glossopharyngeal nerve but also the cranial base of the frill nerve (CN XI).

The vagus nerve goes through the jugular foramen joined by the adornment nerve, both sharing an arachnoid and a dural sheath. Beneath the jugular foramen, the vagus nerve has two augmentations, the prevalent (jugular) and the sub-par (nodose) ganglion, where pseudounipolar neurons are found.

The higher ganglion of the vagus nerve conveys cell assortments of afferent somatosensory neurons. The more significant part of them offers ascent to axons that enter the auricular nerve, a part of the vagus nerve giving real data from the external auditory meatus.

A portion of the fibers structure the meningeal part of the vagus nerve innervating the dura mater in the back cranial fossa, and a few fibers transmit driving forces from the taste receptors in the mucosa of the epiglottis as well as the epiglottic vallecula.

The inferior ganglion of vagus nerve contains collections of real, unique, and general instinctive afferent neurons with axons synapsing halfway in the lone nucleus and their dendrites accepting real data from the larynx, lungs, heart, and the wholesome tract portion starting from the pharynx to the transverse colon.

Cervical piece of the vagus nerve

In the wake of leaving the skull through the jugular foramen, the vagus nerve plunges in the neck secured by the carotid sheath first between the interior carotid supply route and the inner jugular vein, at that point between the regular carotid conduit and the inside jugular vein.

The cervical piece of the vagus nerve radiates four arrangements of branches:

- pharyngeal branches,
- superior laryngeal nerve,
- intermittent laryngeal nerve,
- Cardiovascular branches.

The pharyngeal parts of the vagus nerve emerge from the predominant piece of the second rate vagal ganglion and contain fibers structure the frill nerve (CN XI).

In the neck, the pharyngeal parts of the vagus nerve travel between the outside and inward carotid supply routes to the predominant fringe of the center pharyngeal constrictor, where they convey into a few fibers, which enter parts of the thoughtful chain and glossopharyngeal nerve (CN IX) and partakes in shaping the pharyngeal nerve plexus.

The pharyngeal nerve plexus, together with the frill nerve, innervate every pharyngeal muscle (aside from the stylopharyngeus tissue, that is innervated by the CN IX), mucous layer in the lower some portion of the pharynx, as well as the muscles of the delicate sense of taste (except for the tensor veli palatini tissue, which is innervated by CN V3).

The higher laryngeal nerve is a part of the vagus nerve, which conveys both tactile and engine fibers.

The higher laryngeal nerve emerges from the centerpiece of the inferior ganglion of the vagus nerve and in its course gets a branch from the prevalent cervical thoughtful ganglion, at that point heads out nearby the pharynx to the inner carotid corridor, where it separates into inside and outside parts of the laryngeal nerve.

The inside part of the better laryngeal nerve supplies tangible innervation than the pharynx, yet the outer part of the prevalent laryngeal nerve has engine fibers, which innervate the cricothyroid muscle.

The recurrent laryngeal nerve is a blended part of the vagus nerve containing engine and tactile fibers. The repetitive laryngeal nerve varies in inception and seminar on the left and right side.

The term 'repetitive' demonstrates that they travel the other way to the nerve they branch from. On the left side, the left repetitive laryngeal nerve circles underneath the aortic curve, while the correct nerve circles under the initial segment of the privilege subclavian corridor, in this level, the two nerves give heart fibers to the profound cardiovascular plexus.

After that, the left and right repetitive laryngeal nerves climbs almost a notch between the throat and trachea, near the average surface of the thyroid organ, and afterward enters the lower fringe of the second rate constrictor muscle, entering the larynx.

The engine fiber of the repetitive laryngeal nerve innervates every single laryngeal muscle, except the cricothyroid.

It likewise speaks with the inside laryngeal nerve, providing tactile (afferent) fibers to the laryngeal mucosa under the vocal folds, just as transmitting afferent fibers from the laryngeal stretch receptors.

There are two arrangements of heart branches emerging from the vagus nerve, the second rate, and predominant cervical cardiovascular branches.

The second rate cervical cardiovascular parts of the vagus nerve emerge from the vagus nerve, on the right side.

From the storage compartment of the vagus nerve and the recurrent laryngeal nerve, while on the left side, they emerge from the repetitive nerve as it were.

The second rate cervical cardiovascular branches drop behind the subclavian vein and along the front of the trachea, to join the profound piece of the heart plexus.

The prevalent cervical heart parts of the vagus nerve emerge as two branches from the predominant cervical ganglion.

They run down the neck behind the regular carotid supply route, and before the longus Colli muscle and crosses before the substandard thyroid conduit and the repetitive laryngeal nerve.

The correct branch joins the profound piece of the cardiovascular plexus, while the left branch runs before the left primary carotid vein and over the left half of the curve of the aorta, to join the shallow piece of the heart plexus.

Further, the course of the vagus nerve varies on the two sides. The correct vagus nerve makes a trip back to the jugular vein, crosses the initial segment of the subclavian supply route, and enters the thorax through the predominant thoracic opening.

On the left side, the vagus nerve goes in the thorax in between the left standard corridor and subclavian courses, back to the brachiocephalic vein.

Thoracic piece of the vagus nerve

In the thorax, both the left and also right vagus nerves run behind the pulmonary radix as well as around the centerpiece of the throat, and the fibers combine to frame the esophageal plexus. The mediocre fibers of the esophageal plexus structure the foremost and back vagal trunks.

The front vagal trunk disperses fibers on the first surface of the throat. It comprises basically of fibers from the left vagus.

The back vagal trunk includes fundamentally of fibers from the correct vagus nerve, and they are conveyed on the back surface of the throat.

The two trunks slide through the esophageal rest in the stomach into the stomach cavity.

The abdominal portion of the vagus nerve

In the midriff, the front vagal trunk runs along with the lesser ebb and flow of the stomach where it separates into a few arrangements of branches:

The first gastric branches, which structure the front gastric plexus and supply the stomach; the hepatic branch that moves along with the lesser omentum to the liver, and the celiac branch, which comprises of little branches giving parasympathetic innervation to the celiac nerve plexus.

The back vagal trunk runs along the more prominent ebb and flow of the stomach to the rear surface, where it parts into a few arrangements of branches: the back gastric branches, which structure the front gastric plexus, branches to the kidneys, liver and biliary tract, as well as the celiac branch, which joins the celiac nerve plexus and supplies practically the entirety of the stomach organs.

The vagus nerve capacities add to the autonomic sensory system, which comprises of the parasympathetic and thoughtful parts.

The fundamental patron of the parasympathetic sensory system is the tenth cranial nerve starting from the medulla oblongata in the focal sensory system.

It's the most below piece of the cerebrum and merely sits above where the mind converges into the spinal string.

The vagus is two enormous nerves long fibers made out of numerous littler cells that send data around the body. One develops on the right side of the medulla, another on the left.

In any case, the vast majority allude to both the privilege and left simultaneously when they talk about "the vagus."

Within the medulla, the cell collections of vagal preganglionic neurons are found in the nucleus vague (NA) and the dorsal engine of the vagus (DMV).

These cores supply fibers to the vagus nerve, which rises out of the head, utilizing the jugular foramen. At the degree of the jugular foramen, the superior jugular ganglion of the vagus gives cutaneous branches to the auriculus and outside acoustic meatus.

Only distally, there is a subsequent ganglion, alluded to as the nodose ganglion, gathering tangible innervation from instinctive organs.

The cell assortments of afferent (for example, tactile) neurons are situated in the last ganglion and undertaking to the nucleus of the solitary tract (NTS).

This nucleus transfers contribution to the medulla to control the cardiovascular, respiratory, and gastrointestinal (GI) capacities.

The cervical vagus plummets inside the carotid sheath close by the carotid artery and internal jugular vein. Heart vagal branches leave the cervical vagus and join the cardiovascular plexus.

The left and right repetitive laryngeal nerve, emerging at the degree of the aortic curve and subclavian artery separately, likewise add to the cardiovascular innervation. Other than the heart, the two vagi innervate the lungs through the aspiratory plexus. It contains the accompanying sorts of fibers:

1. Branchial motor; supplying muscles of the pharynx also the larynx.
2. Instinctive sensory; this segment of the vagus nerve is liable for transmitting data from a wide assortment of anatomical destinations, including the heart and lungs, pharynx and larynx, and upper piece of the gastrointestinal tract.
3. Instinctive motor; the inherent engine part conveys parasympathetic fibers from the smooth muscle of the upper respiratory tract, heart, and gastrointestinal tract.
4. Unusual sensory; the unique sensation passed on by the vagus nerve is for taste from the sense of palate and epiglottis.
5. General sensory; the broad tactile segment of the vagus nerve is worried about data from parts of the ear and the Dura inside the back cranial fossa.

The vagus nerve fiber can be named pursues:

- Highly myelinated A fibers, which have low enactment limits
- Lightly myelinated B fibers
- Unmyelinated C fibers, which have high enactment limits.

The B and C fibers have been involved in the guideline of the pulse (19–21). No particular capacity has been ascribed to the vagal A fibers. The recommendation was made that the A fibers may add to the guideline of cytokine discharge.

In concurrence with this plausibility, vagus nerve restraint of cytokine discharge is explicit and can be separated from the vagus nerve guideline of the pulse (Huston, J., unpublished information).

The mitigating cholinergic pathway has a low actuation edge, as would be typical from an A-fiber subordinate channel. Percutaneous incitement of the vagus employing carotid back rub is adequate to repress foundational provocative reactions to endotoxin challenge.

Continuous investigations may depict an immunological-administrative job for the vagus nerve.

Fibers, which are intensely myelinated and accordingly generally touchy to actuation.

Left Vagus Nerve

The left vagus nerve goes in the thorax in between the left regular carotid and left subclavian veins. It proceeds poorly by intersection the aortic curve, where it radiates the huge left repetitive laryngeal nerve.

This nerve circles around the aortic curve from foremost to back, only sidelong to the ligamentum arteriosum. It, at that point, runs superiorly in a score between the throat and trachea (tracheoesophageal groove) to supply eight of the nine laryngeal muscles on the left side.

The central trunk of the vagus nerve proceeds poorly from the curve of the aorta (offering branches to the cardiovascular plexus) and pursues the aorta posteriorly, going behind the foundation of the left lung, where it takes an interest in the pneumonic plexus.

The vagus nerve at that point courses medially and comes to lie on the foremost part of the throat, where it shapes the front oesophagal plexus.

The front oesophagal plexus blends poorly to shape the first vagal trunk. This trunk leaves the thorax by going along the foremost part of the throat through the oesophagal break of the stomach.

Right Vagus Nerve

The correct vagus nerve enters the thorax by the intersection of the privilege subclavian artery. The privilege of the repetitive laryngeal nerve is radiated now.

This nerve circles around the privilege subclavian artery and proceeds superiorly in the right tracheoesophageal section to supply eight of the nine muscles of the larynx on the right side.

The correct vagus nerve proceeds poorly in the thorax, adding to the shallow and profound heart plexuses, and runs back to the base of the right lung. Here it sends a few branches to the back aspiratory plexus.

The correct vagus nerve at that point makes a trip medially to the back part of the throat, where it frames the back oesophagal plexus. The nerves of the back ocsophagal plexus blend to mount the back vagal trunk.

The rear vagal trunk leaves the thorax by going along the back part of the throat through the oesophagal rest of the stomach.

THE SYMPATHETIC AND PARASYMPATHETIC NERVOUS SYSTEM

At the point when you are focused on the thoughtful sensory system makes your body go into an uplifted state regularly alluded to as the "battle or flight reaction."

In this state, pulse increments, bronchial cylinders in your lungs enlarge to take in more oxygen, muscles tense, and more glycogen is changed over into glucose.

This is a naturally preset process to set up the body to flee from things that jeopardize it.

Be that as it may, notwithstanding these littler changes, other body forms are eased back or quit, including salivation creation, gastrointestinal capacity, and absorption.

Even though we may never again need to flee from the things that reason us stress always physically, these progressions to our real capacities still happen.

The vagus nerve is liable for the "quieting" of your body and the returning of the body to homeostasis, otherwise called the "rest and summary" state, after times of pressure.

Subsequently, when the vagus nerve isn't working appropriately, your body doesn't come back to homeostasis as it should.

Huge divisions of the vagus nerve stretch out to the stomach related framework. About 10% to 20% of the vagus nerve cells that interface with the stomach related structure sends directions from the cerebrum to control muscles that move nourishment through the gut.

The development of those muscles is then constrained by a different sensory system implanted inside the dividers of the stomach related framework.

The staying 80% to 90% of the neurons convey factual data from the stomach and digestive organs to the mind.

This correspondence line between the brain and the gastrointestinal tract is known as the cerebrum gut pivot, and it keeps the cerebrum educated about the status of muscle withdrawal, the speed of nourishment entry through the gut, and sentiments of appetite or satiety.

The vagus nerve is so intently laced with the stomach related framework that incitement of the nerve can improve bad tempered gut disorder.

This microbiome speaks with the mind through the vagus nerve, influencing nourishment admission as well as state of mind and irritation reaction.

The real elements of the vagus nerve are classed into two segments:

- Somatic parts: these are sensations felt on the skin or in the muscles.
- Visceral parts: these are sensations felt in the organs of the body.

Tactile elements of the vagus nerve include: giving physical sensation data to the skin behind the ear, the outside piece of the ear channel, and individual pieces of the throat providing instinctive sensation data for the larynx, throat, lungs, trachea, heart.

The vast majority of the stomach-related tract assuming a small job in the vibe of taste neighbouring the base of the tongue

Engine elements of the vagus nerve include: animating muscles in the pharynx, larynx, and the delicate sense of taste, which is the plump zone close the rear of the top of the mouth invigorating muscles in the heart, where it brings down resting pulse animating automatic compressions in the stomach-related tract, including the throat, stomach, and a large portion of the digestion tracts, which enable nourishment to travel through the tract.

Branches

- Auricular nerve
- Pharyngeal nerve
- Superior laryngeal nerve
- Superior cervical cardiovascular parts of the vagus nerve
- Inferior cervical cardiovascular branch
- Recurrent laryngeal nerve
- Thoracic cardiovascular branches
- Tributaries to the pneumonic plexus
- Branches to the oesophagal plexus
- Anterior vagal trunk
- Posterior vagal trunk

- Herring Breuer reflux in alveoli. The vagus runs back to the normal carotid artery and interior jugular vein inside the carotid sheath.

Innervation

Both right and left vagus nerves drop from the mind in the carotid sheath, sidelong to the carotid artery.

The correct vagus nerve offers ascend to the privilege of repetitive laryngeal nerve, which snares around the right subclavian artery and climbs into the neck between the trachea and throat.

The correct vagus at that point crosses anteriorly to the privilege subclavian artery and runs back to the superior vena cava and dives back to the right primary bronchus and adds to cardiovascular, pneumonic, and oesophagal plexuses.

It frames the back vagal trunk at the lower some portion of the throat and enters the stomach through the oesophagal rest. The left vagus nerve goes in the thorax between the left essential carotid artery and left subclavian artery and slides on the aortic curve.

It offers to ascend to one side repetitive laryngeal nerve, which snares around the aortic curve to one side of the ligamentum arteriosum and rises between the trachea and throat.

The left vagus further radiates thoracic cardiovascular branches, separates into pneumonic plexus, proceeds into the oesophagal plexus, and enters the stomach area as the first vagal trunk in the oesophagal break of the stomach.

The vagus nerve supplies engine parasympathetic fibers to every one of the organs except for the suprarenal (adrenal) organs, starting from the neck to the second section of the transverse colon. The vagus additionally controls a couple of skeletal muscles, to be specific:

- Cricothyroid muscle
- Levator veli palatini muscle
- Salpingopharyngeus muscle
- Palatoglossus muscle
- Palatopharyngeus muscle
- Superior, center and second rate pharyngeal constrictors
- Muscles of the larynx (discourse).

This implies the vagus nerve is liable for such fluctuated assignments as pulse, gastrointestinal peristalsis, sweating, and many muscle developments in the mouth.

Including discourse (employing the recurrent laryngeal nerve) and keeping the larynx open for breathing (through the activity of the back cricoarytenoid muscle, the primary abductor of the vocal folds).

It likewise has some afferent fibers that innervate the inward (waterway) segment of the external ear, through the Auricular branch (otherwise called Alderman's nerve) and part of the meninges.

This clarifies why an individual may hack when tickled on their ear (for example, when attempting to evacuate ear wax with a cotton swab).

The vagus nerve and the heart

Parasympathetic innervation of the heart is intervened by the vagus nerve. In particular, the vagus nerve acts to bring down the pulse.

The correct vagus innervates the sinoatrial hub. Parasympathetic hyperstimulation inclines those influenced to bradyarrhythmias. The left vagus, when hyperstimulated, inclines the heart to atrioventricular (AV) squares.

In this area, neuroscientist Otto Loewi previously demonstrated that nerves discharge substances called synapses, which have impacts on receptors in target tissues.

Loewi depicted the substance discharged by the vagus nerve as vagus stuff, which was later seen as acetylcholine. The vagus nerve has three cores in the CNS related to cardiovascular control, the dorsal engine nucleus, the nucleus ambiguus, and the single nucleus.

The parasympathetic yield to the heart comes mostly from neurons in the nucleus ambiguus and, to a lesser degree, from the dorsal engine nucleus.

The single nucleus gets a real contribution to the condition of the cardiovascular framework, being an integrational center for the baroreflex. Medications that repress the muscarinic cholinergic receptor (anticholinergics, for example, atropine and scopolamine) are called vagolytic because they restrain the activity of the vagus nerve on the heart, gastrointestinal tract and different organs.

Anticholinergic medications increment pulse and are utilized to treat bradycardia (slow pulse) and asystole, which is the point at which the heart has no electrical action.

The capacity of Vagus Nerve

The part of Vagus in the Functions of the Autonomic Nervous System, close by the thoughtful sensory system and the enteric sensory system (ENS), the parasympathetic sensory system speaks to one of the three parts of the autonomic sensory system.

The meaning of thoughtful and parasympathetic sensory systems is primarily anatomical. The vagus nerve is the principal supporter of the parasympathetic sensory system. The other three parasympathetic cranial nerves are nervus oculomotorius, the nervus facialis, and the nervus glossopharyngeus.

The most significant capacity of the vagus nerve is afferent, bringing data of the inward organs, for example, gut, liver, heart, and lungs to the mind.

This proposes the internal organs are significant wellsprings of real data to the cerebrum. The stomach as the most prominent surface toward the external world and might, along these lines, is an especially significant tactile organ.

Verifiably, the vagus has been examined as an efferent nerve and as an adversary of the thoughtful sensory system.

Most organs get parasympathetic efferents through the vagus nerve and thoughtful efferents through the splanchnic nerves. Together with the reflective sensory systems, the parasympathetic sensory system is answerable for the guideline of vegetative capacities by acting contrary to one another.

The parasympathetic innervation causes dilatation of veins and bronchioles and incitement of salivary organs. Despite what might be expected, the thoughtful innervation prompts a narrowing of veins, a dilatation of bronchioles, an expansion in pulse, and a tightening of intestinal and urinary sphincters.

In the gastrointestinal tract, the actuation of the parasympathetic sensory system builds inside motility and glandular discharge.

Rather than it, the thoughtful action prompts a decrease of intestinal movement and a reduction of bloodstream to the gut, permitting a higher bloodstream to the heart and the muscles, when the individual faces existential pressure.

The ENS emerges from neural peak cells of the vagal source and comprises of a nerve plexus installed in the intestinal divider, stretching out over the entire gastrointestinal tract from the throat to the butt.

It is evaluated that the human ENS contains around 100–500 million neurons.

This is the most significant aggregation of nerve cells in the human body. Since the ENS is like the mind in regards to structure, capacity, and concoction coding, it has been depicted as "the subsequent cerebrum" or "the cerebrum inside the gut."

It comprises of two ganglionated plexuses—the submucosal plexus, which manages gastrointestinal bloodstream and controls the epithelial cell capacities and emission and the myenteric plexus, which chiefly directs the unwinding and withdrawal of the intestinal divider.

The ENS fills in as an inner boundary and controls the major enteric procedures, for example, safe reaction, distinguishing supplements, motility, microvascular flow, and epithelial emission of liquids, particles, and bioactive peptides.

There is "correspondence" between the vagal nerve and the ENS, and the first transmitter is cholinergic initiation through nicotinic receptors. Cooperation of ENS and the vagal nerve as a piece of the CNS prompts a bidirectional progression of data.

Then again, the ENS in the little and substantial inside additionally can work very free of vagal control as it entails full reflex circuits, including tactile neurons and engine neurons.

They direct muscle action and motility, liquid transitions, mucosal bloodstream, and mucosal hindrance work. ENS neurons are likewise in close contact to cells of the versatile and inborn resistant framework and direct their capacities and exercises.

Maturing and cell misfortune in the ENS are related to grumblings, for example, stoppage, incontinence, and departure issue.

The loss of the ENS in the little and digestive organ might be dangerous (Hirschsprung's illness; intestinal pseudo-hindrance), while the loss of the vagal nerve in these regions isn't. Vagus Nerve as a Link connecting the Central and ENS

The association between the CNS and the ENS additionally alluded to as the mind-gut hub empowers the bidirectional association between the cerebrum and the gastrointestinal tract.

It is liable for observing the physiological homeostasis and interfacing the passionate and subjective zones of the mind with fringe intestinal capacities, for example, safe enactment, intestinal porousness, enteric reflex, and enteroendocrine flagging.

This cerebrum gut pivot incorporates the mind, the spinal rope, the autonomic sensory system (thoughtful, parasympathetic, and ENS), and the hypothalamic-pituitary-adrenal (HPA) hub.

The vagal efferent sends the sign "down" from the cerebrum to gut through efferent fibers, which represent 10–20% all things considered and the vagal afferents "up" from the intestinal divider to the mind representing 80–90% everything being equal.

The vagal afferent pathways are engaged with the enactment/guideline of the HPA hub, which organizes the versatile reactions of the creature to stressors of any sort.

Environmental worry, just as raised foundational genius provocative cytokines, initiates the HPA hub through the emission of the corticotrophin-discharging factor (CRF) from the nerve center.

The CRF discharge invigorates adrenocorticotropic hormone (ACTH) emission from the pituitary organ. This incitement, thus, prompts cortisol discharge from the adrenal organs.

Cortisol is a significant pressure hormone that influences numerous human organs, including the mind, bones, muscles, and muscle versus fat.

Both neural (vagus) and hormonal (HPA pivot) lines of correspondence consolidate to enable the mind to impact the exercises of intestinal useful effector cells, for example, insusceptible cells, the epithelial cells, enteric neurons, smooth muscle cells, the interstitial cells of Cajal, and also enterochromaffin cells.

These cells, then again, are affected by the gut small scale biota.

The gut smaller scale biota importantly affects the cerebrum gut pivot collaborating locally with intestinal cells and ENS, yet additionally by legitimately impacting neuroendocrine and metabolic frameworks.

Developing information bolsters the job of miniaturized scale biota in affecting tension and burdensome like practices. Studies led on without germ creatures showed that small scale biota impact pressure reactivity and nervousness like conduct and direct the set point for HPA movement.

Accordingly, these creatures, for the most part, show a diminished nervousness and an expanded pressure reaction with increased degrees of ACTH and cortisol.

If there comes an occurrence of nourishment input, vagal afferents innervating the gastrointestinal tract give a fast and discrete record of absorbable nourishment just as coursing and put away powers, while vagal efferents together with the hormonal instruments codetermine the pace of supplement ingestion, stockpiling, and preparation.

Histological and electrophysiological proof demonstrates that instinctive afferent endings of the vagus nerve in the digestive tract express various exhibits of substance and mechanosensitive receptors.

These receptors are focuses on gut hormones and regulatory peptides that are discharged from enteroendocrine cells of the gastrointestinal framework in light of supplements, by distension of the stomach and by a neuronal sign.

They impact the control of nourishment admission and guideline of satiety, gastric discharging, and vitality balance by transmitting signals emerging from the upper gut to the nucleus of the single tract in the cerebrum.

The vast majority of these hormones, for example, peptide cholecystokinin (CCK), ghrelin, and leptin are touchy to the supplement content in the gut and are engaged with directing momentary sentiments of appetite and satiety.

Cholecystokinin directs gastrointestinal capacities, including hindrance of gastric discharging and nourishment admission through the enactment of CCK-1 receptors on vagal afferent fibers exciting the gut.

Furthermore, CCK is significant for the discharge of pancreatic liquid and creating gastric corrosive, getting the gallbladder, diminishing gastric exhausting, and encouraging absorption. Immersed fat, long-chain unsaturated fats, amino acids, and small peptides that outcome from protein assimilation invigorates the arrival of CCK from the small digestive system.

There are different naturally dynamic types of CCK, arranged by the quantity of amino acids in them, i.e., CCK-5, CCK-8, CCK-22, and CCK-33.

In neurons, CCK-8 is consistently the prevailing structure, though the endocrine gut cells contain a blend of small and more significant CCK peptides of which CCK-33 or CCK-22 frequently prevails.

In rodents, both long-and short-chain unsaturated fats from nourishment enact jejunal vagal afferent nerve fibers, yet do as such by particular systems.

Short-chain unsaturated fats, for example, butyric acid directly affect vagal afferent terminals while the long-chain unsaturated fats initiate vagal afferents through a CCK-subordinate system.

The exogenous organization of CCK seems to hinder endogenous CCK discharge. CCK is likewise present in enteric vagal afferent neurons, in the cerebral cortex, in the thalamus, nerve center, basal ganglia, and dorsal hindbrain, and capacities as a synapse.

It legitimately initiates vagal afferent terminals in the NTS by expanding calcium discharge.

Further, there is proof that CCK can actuate neurons in the hindbrain and myenteric intestinal plexus (a plexus which gives engine innervation to the two layers of the active layer of the gut), in rodents and that vagotomy or capsaicin treatment brings about a weakening of CCK-initiated Fo's articulation (a kind of a proto-oncogene) in the mind.

There is likewise generous proof that raised degrees of CCK actuate sentiments of nervousness. Subsequently, CCK is utilized as a test specialist to show nervousness issues in people and creatures.

Ghrelin is another hormone discharged into the course from the stomach and assumes a key job in animating nourishment consumption by repressing vagal afferent terminating.

Flowing ghrelin levels are expanded by fasting and fall after a feast. Focal or fringe organization of acylated ghrelin to rodents intensely invigorates nourishment admission and development hormone discharge, and constant organization causes weight gain.

The activity of ghrelin's on sustaining is cancelled or weakened in rodents that have experienced vagotomy or treatment with capsaicin, a particular afferent neurotoxin. In people, intravenous imbuement or subcutaneous infusion increments the two sentiments of appetite and nourishment consumption, since ghrelin smothers insulin discharge.

Consequently, it isn't surprising that emission is upset in stoutness and insulin obstruction.

Leptin receptors have likewise been recognized in the vagus nerve. Concentrates in rodents demonstrate that leptin and CCK interface synergistically to initiate momentary restraint of nourishment allow and prolonged haul decrease of body weight.

The epithelial cells that react to both ghrelin and leptin are situated close to the vagal mucosal endings and balance the movement of vagal afferents, acting in the show to manage nourishment admission.

In the wake of fasting and diet-prompted obesity in mice, leptin loses its potentiating impact on vagal mucosal afferents.

The gastrointestinal tract is the critical interface among nourishment and the human body and can detect essential preferences for similarly as the tongue, using comparative G-protein-coupled taste receptors.

Diverse taste characteristics actuate the arrival of various gastric peptides. Harsh taste receptors can be considered as potential focuses to lessen hunger by invigorating the appearance of CCK.

Further, initiation of unpleasant taste receptors invigorates ghrelin emission and, along these lines, influences the vagus nerve.

VN as Modulator of Intestinal Immune Homeostasis

The gastrointestinal tract is continually faced with nourishment antigens, potential pathogens, and beneficial intestinal microbiota that present a hazard factor for intestinal irritation. It is profoundly innervated by vagal fibers that associate the

CNS with the intestinal insusceptible framework, making vagus a significant part, the neuroendocrine-invulnerable pivot. This pivot is engaged with composed neural, conduct, and endocrine reactions, vital for the chief line guard against irritation.

For instance, because of pathogens and different damaging boosts, tumour-putrefaction factor-alpha (TNF-α), a cytokine, is created by enacted macrophages, dendritic cells, and different cells in the mucosa.

Together with prostaglandins and interferons, TNF-α is a significant go-between of the neighbourhood and foundational aggravation and builds cause the cardinal clinical indications of irritation, including heat, growing torment, and redness. Counter-administrative components, for example, immunologically skilful cells and mitigating cytokines, typically limit the intense provocative reaction and avoid the spread of incendiary go-between into the circulatory system.

Further, there is a "hard-wired" association between the anxious and safe framework that works as a calming component.

The dorsal vagal complex, involving the physical cores of the single tract, the territory postrema, and the dorsal engine nucleus of the vagus, reacts to expanded, flowing measures of TNF-α by adjusting engine movement in the vagus nerve.

The mitigating limits of the vagus nerve intercede through three distinct pathways.

The primary pathway is the HPA pivot, which has been portrayed previously.

The subsequent pathway is the splenic thoughtful calming pathway, where the vagus nerve invigorates the thoughtful splenic nerve.

Norepinephrine (NE) (noradrenaline) discharged at the distal finish of the splenic nerve connects to the β2 adrenergic receptor of splenic lymphocytes that ejects ACh.

At last, ACh hinders the arrival of TNF-α by spleen macrophages through α-7-nicotinic ACh receptors. The previous pathway, called the cholinergic calming pathway (CAIP), is interceded through vagal efferent fibers that neurotransmitter onto enteric neurons, which thus discharge ACh at the synaptic intersection with macrophages. ACh ties to α-7-nicotinic ACh receptors of those macrophages to restrain the TNF-α.

Contrasted with the HPA hub, the CAIP has one of a kind property, for example, a rapid neural conductance, which empowers a quick modulatory contribution to the influenced area of irritation.

Like this, the CAIP assumes a pivotal job in the visceral resistant reaction and homeostasis and presents an exceptionally intriguing objective for the advancement of novel medications for incendiary maladies identified with the gut invulnerable framework.

The irritation detecting and aggravation smothering capacities sketched out above give the chief segments of the incendiary reflex.

The presence of pathogenic living beings enacts intrinsic safe cells that discharge cytokines. These this way, actuate tangible fibers that arise in the vagus nerve to the neurotransmitter in the nucleus tractus solitarius.

Expanded efferent flag in the vagus nerve stifles fringe cytokine discharge through macrophage nicotinic receptors and the CAIP. Along these lines, trial enactment of the CAIP by direct electrical incitement of the efferent vagus nerve hinders the combination of TNF-α in the liver, spleen, and heart and weakens serum convergences of TNF-α.

All the more distally, the left and right vagus run with the throat through the diaphragmatic break. After entering the stomach pit, the left and right vagus become the foremost and back vagus, separately.

Notwithstanding, one needs to remember that every trunk gets fibers from both cervical vagus nerves. The quantity of back and foremost trunks going through the diaphragmatic opening is variable, up to two in the previous and three in the last mentioned.

The front trunk appropriates gastric branches to the foremost part of the stomach and emits a hepatic branch. Other than innervating the liver, the hepatic stem emits branches to the pylorus and the proximal piece of the duodenum and pancreas.

Then again, the back trunk disperses one gastric branch to the proximal back part of the stomach and also another one to the coeliac plexus, which innervates the spleen and GI tract coming to the extent the left colonic flexure.

The internal organ gets extra parasympathetic innervation through the pelvic splanchnic nerve, which ends in the pelvic plexus and develops as the colonic and rectal nerve.

The afferent vagus nerve impels the GI tract utilizing vagal terminals both in the lamina propria and in the muscular outside. In any case, the efferent vagus nerve fibers connect with neurons of the enteric sensory system (ENS).

The ENS comprises a thick meshwork of nerve fibers arranged in the submucosal (for example, submucosal plexus) and outside solid compartment of the digestive system (for instance, myenteric plexus).

By methods for electrophysiological and anterograde tracer examines, it was demonstrated that preganglionic parasympathetic fibers (for example, both vagal and sacral innervation) legitimately connect with numerous postganglionic myenteric neurons by the development of varicosities, though scarcely any vagal fibers speak with submucosal neurons.

The preganglionic innervation of the GI tract shows a run of the mill rostrocaudal inclination with the most elevated thickness of innervated myenteric neurons in the stomach and duodenum pursued by a progressive decrease in the small digestive system and colon.

The way that gastric myenteric neurons are enacted by vagal info was additionally demonstrated immunohistochemically with the identification of c-Fos and phosphorylated c-AMP reaction component restricting protein (p-CREB), which are markers for neuronal action.

The particular area of every terminal has connections with its physiological capacity.

Maybe the best hugeness of the vagus nerve is that it is the body's significant parasympathetic nerve, providing parasympathetic fibers to all the vital organs of the head, neck, chest, and midriff.

The vagus nerve is answerable for the gag reflex (and the hack reflex when the ear trench is invigorated), easing back the pulse, controlling perspiring, managing circulatory strain, animating peristalsis of the gastrointestinal tract, and controlling vascular tone.

It mediates in numerous capacities, from mouth developments to heartbeat, and in like manner, when influenced, it can cause different side effects.

FUNCTIONS OF VAGUS NERVE

A portion of the vagus nerve works in our body are:

– It directs heartbeat, controls muscle developments, and keeps up the pace of relaxing.

– It keeps up the working of the stomach related tract, permitting the constriction of the stomach and digestive system muscles to process nourishment.

– Facilitates unwinding after an unpleasant circumstance or shows that we are in threat, and we don't need to bring down the watchman.

–Send real data to the cerebrum about organ status.

Additionally clarified beneath are a more significant amount of its capacities.

The Vagus Nerve Prevents Inflammation.

A specific measure of aggravation after damage or sickness is typical. In any case, an excess is connected to numerous illnesses and conditions, from sepsis to the immune system condition rheumatoid joint pain. The vagus nerve operates an extensive system of fibers positioned like covert operatives around the entirety of your organs.

At the point when it gets a sign for nascent aggravation—the nearness of cytokines or a substance called tumor putrefaction factor (TNF) cautions the mind and draws out calming synapses that direct the body's immune reaction.

It Helps You Take Memories.

A University of Virginia study in rodents indicated that animating their vagus nerves reinforced their memory. The activity discharged the synapse norepinephrine into the amygdala, which solidified recollections. Related examinations were done in people, proposing promising medications for conditions like Alzheimer's ailment.

IT HELPS YOU BREATHE.

The synapse acetylcholine, evoked by the vagus nerve, advises your lungs to relax. It's one reason that Botox—frequently utilized cosmetically—can be possibly risky because it intrudes on your acetylcholine generation.

You can be that as it may likewise invigorate your vagus nerve by doing stomach breathing or holding your breath for up to four to eight rounds.

It's intimately involved with your heart.

The vagus nerve is answerable for controlling the pulse through electrical driving forces to particular muscle tissue—the heart's natural pacemaker—in the correct chamber, where acetylcholine discharge eases back the beat.

By estimating the time between your heart pulsates and afterwards plotting this on an outline over the long run, specialists can decide your pulse fluctuation or HRV. This information can offer signs about the versatility of your heart and vagus nerve.

It initiates your body's relaxation response.

When your ever-cautious thoughtful sensory system fires up the battle or flight reactions—pouring the pressure hormone cortisol and adrenaline in the body—the vagus nerve advises your body to relax by discharging acetylcholine.

The vagus nerve's ringlets stretch out to numerous organs, acting like fibre-optic links that send guidelines to discharge chemicals and proteins like prolactin, vasopressin, and oxytocin, which quiet you down.

Individuals with a more grounded vagus reaction might be bound to recoup all the more rapidly after pressure, damage, or disease.

It translates between the gut and brain.

Your gut utilises the vagus nerve like a walkie-talkie to tell your cerebrum how you're feeling utilizing electric motivations called "activity possibilities." Your gut emotions are genuine.

Over-stimulation of the vagus nerve is the most common cause of fainting.

If you tremble or get nauseous at seeing blood or while getting an influenza shot, you're not powerless. You're encountering "vagal syncope." Your body, reacting to pressure, overstimulates the vagus nerve, causing your circulatory strain and pulse to drop.

During outrageous syncope, the bloodstream is confined to your cerebrum, and you lose awareness. In any case, more often than not, you need to sit or rests for the side effects of dying down.

The electrical stimulation of the vagus nerve diminishes inflammation and may inhibit it altogether.

Neurosurgeon Kevin Tracey was the foremost to show that invigorating the vagus nerve can fundamentally lessen the irritation. Results on rodents were so effective, and he replicated the investigation in people with shocking outcomes.

The formation of inserts to invigorate the vagus nerve utilizing electronic inserts indicated a marked decrease and even reduction in rheumatoid joint pain—which has no known fix and is frequently treated with the dangerous medications—hemorrhagic stun, and other similarly genuine provocative disorders.

Vagus nerve stimulation has developed a new field of medicine.

Prodded on by the accomplishment of vagal nerve incitement to treat irritation and epilepsy, a prospering field of restorative investigation, known as bioelectronics, might be the eventual fate of medication.

Utilizing inserts that convey electric motivations to different body parts, researchers and specialists would like to treat disease with fewer meds and fewer symptoms.

VAGUS NERVE TESTING

To test the vagus nerve, a specialist may check the gag reflex. During this piece of the assessment, the specialist may utilize a delicate cotton swab to tickle the rear of the throat on the two sides.

This should make the individual gag. On the off chance that the individual doesn't gag, this might be because of an issue with the vagus nerve.

Vagus nerve issues

Nerve Harm

Harm to the vagus nerve could have a scope of manifestations because the nerve is so long and influences numerous zones.

Potential side effects of harm to the vagus nerve include:

- Difficulty talking or loss of voice
- A voice that is raspy or wheezy
- Trouble drinking fluids
- Failure of the gag reflex
- Pain in the ear
- Unusual pulse
- Abnormal pulse
- decreased generation of stomach corrosive
- Nausea or heaving

- Abdominal swelling or agony

The indications somebody may have relied upon what some portion of the nerve is harmed.

Gastroparesis

Specialists accept that harm to the vagus nerve may likewise cause a condition called gastroparesis.

This condition influences the automated constrictions of the stomach related framework, which keeps the stomach from appropriately discharging.

Side effects of gastroparesis include:

- Nausea or regurgitating, particularly retching undigested nourishment hours in the wake of eating
- Loss of hunger or feeling full soon after beginning a dinner
- Acid reflux
- Abdominal torment or swelling
- Unexplained weight reduction
- Fluctuations in glucose

A few people make gastroparesis in the wake of experiencing a vagotomy strategy, which evacuates all or part of the vagus nerve.

Vasovagal syncope

Now and again the vagus nerve blows up to specific pressure triggers, for example,

- exposure to extraordinary warmth
- fear of real mischief
- During seeing blood or having blood drawn
- straining, including attempting to having a stable discharge
- standing for quite a while

Keep in mind, and the vagus nerve animates specific muscles in the heart that help to slow pulse.

At the point when it overcompensates, it can cause an unexpected drop in pulse and circulatory strain, bringing about swooning. This is known as vasovagal syncope.

The Potential Effects Of Vagus Nerve Dysfunction

Numerous people with vagus nerve brokenness know uneasiness just as discouragement from synapse uneven characters.

Different side effects may incorporate supplement insufficiencies (especially B nutrients), insulin dysregulation, equalization or coordination issues, strange pulse, narrow mindedness to development or movement ailment, gastrointestinal problems, exhaustion, poor memory or center, diminished processing, liver brokenness, trouble gulping or breathing, swooning, and so forth.

Luckily, your professional can run tests and help execute ways to direct the vagus nerve. The vagus nerve brokenness manifestations that are being shown can help your sustenance specialist decide the precise healthful mediations that might be actualized for your customized administration convention.

Note that you ought not to begin any eating regimen or supplementation convention without talking about any progressions with your expert.

Signs and Symptoms of Vagus Nerve Dysfunction

Given the broad associations between the cerebrum and gut utilizing the vagus nerve and its branches, there are various areas helpless against brokenness. These districts can be assembled into three primary zones:

- Communication inside the cerebrum
- The connection from the cerebrum to different organs
- Communication from different organs to the cerebrum

Contingent upon which territory is beset, vagus nerve brokenness may show as:

- Aggression
- Anxiety
- Brain haze
- Chronic irritation
- Delayed stomach exhausting
- Depression
- Difficulty gulping
- Dizziness or blacking out
- Fatigue
- Heart rate changes (significant or low)
- Heartburn
- Irritable Bowel Syndrome (IBS)
- Vitamin B12 inadequacy
- Weight gain

Left undiscovered or untreated, vagus nerve brokenness can prompt progressively genuine maladies including:

- Alcohol dependence
- Autism
- Bulimia
- Cancer
- Chronic cardiovascular breakdown
- Fibromyalgia
- Heart infection
- Leaky Gut Syndrome
- Memory issue or Alzheimer's infection
- Migraines
- Mood issue
- Multiple Sclerosis (MS)
- Obesity

- Obsessive-Compulsive Disorder (OCD)
- Poor blood course
- Tinnitus

Staying away from illnesses and way of life decisions that harm the Vagus Nerve is fundamental to keeping the above signs and indications under control. These incorporate liquor abuse, tension, and diabetes, and exhaustion, physical harm to the Vagus Nerve, weak stance, and stress.

Vagus Nerve Disorder

A solid vagus nerve underpins your stomach related framework, serves to manage your rest examples, and quiets down your nerves.

Figuring out how to control vagal tone is related to a decrease in aggravation and better visualization in individuals experiencing incessant ailment, headaches, auto-save issues, uneasiness, and wretchedness.

The vagus nerve issue is mainly separated into two classes. There are the scatters that are brought about by a nerve that is underactive or not working appropriately, and there are those that are brought about by your vagus nerve, exaggerating to the boosts it gets.

An underactive vagus nerve can prompt a condition called gastroparesis. This condition prompts sickness, indigestion, stomach torments, fits in the stomach, and weight reduction because of the stomach related framework having excessively little of the synthetic substances it needs to separate nourishment.

An underactive vagus nerve can likewise prompt a dropping pulse. Pacemakers can be utilized to help keep up a vibration that is beneficial to help avert the pulse from dropping to an unsafe level and causing risky conditions, for example, a trance-like state.

Overactive vagus nerves can cause visit blacking out. All alone, this isn't especially dangerous. However, this can prompt wounds when an individual falls because of the quick loss of awareness.

Side effects of a vagus nerve issue will fluctuate dependent on whether the nerve is under or over responding to upgrades.

One of the most well-known symptoms of this issue is torment, which will feel fundamentally the same as a squeezed nerve. This torment may likewise be coupled by muscle cramps when you move or perform an activity, for example, getting objects. In extreme cases, this agony can make it hard to walk appropriately.

You may likewise experience difficulty gulping because the vagus nerve additionally controls the muscles that take into account the admission of nourishment. You may also see that your gag reflex is never again as dynamic when the vagus nerve is harm.

You may likewise see that your voice is adjusted because of the muscles in the throat, responding unexpectedly.

Notwithstanding the organ harm or challenges that go with a harmed vagus nerve, there are opposite reactions that might be an indication that your vagus nerve isn't working appropriately.

You might be progressively powerless to creating peptic ulcers because the body is delivering more stomach corrosive than it should. You may likewise start to create blockage because your digestion tracts are not directing water admission how they should.

Patients who are managing an irregular vagus nerve may experience issues controlling their pee and may experience the ill effects of urinary incontinence.

Nervousness

At the point when we are exposed to upsetting circumstances, the thoughtful sensory system is actuated. If the pressure perseveres and we can't kill the physiological reaction that triggers it, it won't sit back before issues show up.

At the cerebrum level, this includes the initiation of two pathways: the nerve center pituitary-adrenal hub and the mind digestive tract hub.

The cerebrum reacts to pressure and tension by expanding the generation of hormones (CRFs) that movement from the nerve center to the pituitary organ where they instigate the arrival of another hormone (ACTH), which like this ventures out through the circulation system to the adrenal organs to invigorate cortisol and adrenaline enlistment.

Which go about as invulnerable framework silencers and incendiary antecedents, which is the reason when we feel focused, and on edge, we get sick effectively and, eventually, we can wind up experiencing grief, a turmoil which has been connected to a fiery mind reaction.

What's more, as though that were insufficient, continuous pressure and tension reason an expansion in glutamate in the cerebrum, a synapse that, when created in abundance, causes headache, discouragement, and uneasiness.

Likewise, a significant level of cortisol lessens the volume of the hippocampus, the piece of the cerebrum answerable for the development of new recollections.

The inclusion of the vagus nerve will prompt side effects, for example, tipsiness, gastrointestinal issues, arrhythmias, trouble in breathing, and lopsided enthusiastic reactions.

Truth be told, as the vagus nerve can't initiate the unwinding signal, the thoughtful sensory system keeps dynamic, this will make the individual react rashly and experience the ill effects of uneasiness.

It is likewise curious that an examination created at the University of Miami found that the vagal tone is transmitted from mother to youngster.

Ladies experiencing nervousness, wretchedness, or encountering a lot of outrage during pregnancy had a lower vagal movement, and their youngsters additionally displayed little vagal action and lower levels of dopamine and serotonin.

Despondency

Vagus nerve incitement has been utilized to treat despair just lately. Research on how well it functions is as yet progressing. It's commonly viewed if all else fails alternative. Specialists, as a rule, suggest that you attempt various sorts and mixes of medicine and psychotherapy before attempting VNS.

The treatment is prescribed for grown-ups 18 and more established who have treatment-safe discouragement. The FDA additionally mandates that you proceed with different types of treatment-related to VNS. Different medicines incorporate drug and social psychological treatment.

Individuals who are pregnant or have some other neurological condition probably won't be qualified for VNS.

Your primary care specialist can assist you in deciding if vagus nerve incitement is a possibility for you. Numerous medical coverage plans don't cover VNS.

Vagus nerve incitement includes a significant medical procedure to embed the beat generator. Difficulties may emerge both during and after a medical procedure. Usual dangers related to the medical system include:

- Infection
- Pain
- Breathing issues
- Damage to the vagus nerve

Another hazard with VNS medical procedure is the plausibility of vocal string loss of motion. This can happen if the gadget moves after implantation.

You may likewise need to quit taking certain drugs a few days before the strategy.

Individuals who have had VNS medical procedures may encounter an assortment of symptoms a while later. These can include:

- Chest torment
- Throat torment
- Difficulty gulping
- Difficulty relaxing

Despondency may likewise exacerbate in specific individuals. The beat generator may break or should be balanced at times, requiring another medical procedure.

Intestinal Problems

Vagal fibers are anticipated all through the gastrointestinal (GI) tract and connect with the gut to direct nourishment admission, absorption, hindrance keeping, and insusceptibility.

Nourishment consumption prompts satiety through the initiation of a few pathways: the arrival of different peptides from enteroendocrine cells (EEC), the immediate activity of specific supplements, and mechanoreceptor incitement because of gastric distension.

Most afferent vagal endings in mucosal lamina propria are believed to be chemoreceptors detecting the nearness of hormones, peptides, and supplements discharged by epithelial and neuroendocrine cells.

Conversely, the terminal vagal structures in the outside muscle layers and the myenteric plexus are viewed as mechanoreceptors identifying GI distension.

These tactile signs are transferred to the NTS, where the afferent data is prepared. Proper vagal efferent yield is transmitted from the DMV.

The last has a significant metabolic and dietary capacity since the electrical incitement of DMV prompts an expanded emission of gastric corrosive insulin and glucagon.

Besides, the discharge of gastric corrosive, insulin, glucagon, and pancreatic polypeptide is additionally raised when the fringe vagus nerve is animated.

These reactions are altogether annulled by vagotomy, organization of atropine, or hexamethonium. Other than its dietary and metabolic capacities, the vagus nerve likewise has impacts on the intestinal obstruction work through insusceptible cells (for example, pole cells) and the actuation of enteric glial cells through the ENS.

Dietary Intake and Metabolism Regulation Chemical incitement.

The EECs react to supplement detecting in the lumen by the basolateral discharge of leptin in the stomach and cholecystokinin (CCK) in the small digestive system.

Tracer considers indicated that EECs lie in close region to mucosal vagal afferent terminals anticipating from the nodose ganglia using the myenteric plexus.

The nearby anatomical situation between vagal afferents and EECs empowers CCK and leptin to go about as paracrine factors, which initiate CCK-A26 and Ob-R receptors communicated on afferent fibers, separately.

Electrophysiological considers you have affirmed these anatomical perceptions since CCK invigorates afferent nerve.

This afferent flagging is additionally handed-off to the NTS. Synergistic vagal actuation by CCK and leptin prompt restraint of nourishment consumption.

What's more, CCK alone represses gastric purging and invigorates biliary and pancreatic emission.

Afferent vagal fibers get data from the inward milieu of the GI tract using mechanical flagging and concoction (for example, enteroendocrine hormone discharge and certain nourishment supplements) and immunological incitement (for example pro-inflammatory cytokines).

This tangible data is transmitted to the nucleus of the single tract (NTS) to mount a proper efferent (for example engine) reaction through the dorsal engine nucleus of the vagus (DMV, for example, the discharge of neuroendocrine hormones and varieties in GI motility, boundary capacity, and adjustment of the intestinal insusceptible reaction.

Efferent Vagus Nerve

DMVNTS A B

Afferent Vagus Nerve

Motility

Barrier function

Discharge Anti-provocative

CCK

Leptin Lipids

Distension

Cytokines

Afferent Vagus Nerve

Motility Distension

CCK

Lipids

Leptin

Cytokines

Discharge

Calming

Hindrance work

Afferent Vagus Nerve

For sure, the organization of specific CCK-A receptors opponents preceding a dinner expands nourishment ingestion and gastric discharging, however, hinders pancreatic emission.

These impacts of CCK are subject to a flawless vagal stockpile since vagotomy or pulverization of little distance across vagal afferent C fibers by capsaicin cancels the activities of CCK.

Mechanical incitement besides chemosensory signal transduction, the afferent curve of the vagus is likewise actuated by gastric distension through the instigation of afferent vagal mechanoreceptor in the GI tract.

Two applicant mechanoreceptors of the vagus nerve have been portrayed: the intraganglionic laminar consummation (IGLE) and intramuscular clusters (IMAs).

The previous terminal comprises of totals of terminal puncta related to myenteric neurons just as connective tissue structures encompassing the myenteric ganglia. IGLEs are unarguably the densest in the stomach and become inadequate all the more caudally.

The nearby anatomical closeness between the connective tissue layers and the ganglia shows that IGLEs can recognize the shearing powers between the symmetrical muscle layers.

Electrophysiological thinks about affirm that IGLE could go about as low edge strain receptors since twisting of the stomach prompts enactment of pressure touchy vagal mechanoreceptors.

An inferior of noticeable vagal mechanoreceptors are IMAs, which comprise of parallel varieties of neurite terminals coursing parallel to muscle packages in the longitudinal or round muscle layers and lie in the neighbouring region of interstitial cells of Cajal (ICC).

IMAs are generally situated in the upper stomach, lower oesophagal and pyloric sphincters. In light of the morphological highlights, IMAs seems to go about as stretch receptors delicate to shearing powers in the long hub.

Be that as it may, electrophysiological thinks about have not had the option to decide the genuine usefulness of IMAs unambiguously.

The tangible vagal mechanoreceptors invigorated by gastric distension, are the principal trigger of vago-vagal reflexes, for example, gastric settlement, restraint of nourishment consumption, and antral peristalsis.

Distension likewise seems to act in cooperative energy with CCK to expand the afferent movement and subsequently decline nourishment admission.

Nonetheless, Grundy et al. differ in the way that CCK applies an immediate impact on vagal afferent mechanoreceptors. Instead, they recommend that the activity of CCK is intervened through the tactile vagal chemoreceptors in the mucosa. The Vagus Nerve as Intestinal Barrier Keeper :

Intestinal epithelial cells keep up an exacting boundary between the outer and inner conditions employing the statement of tight intersections.

The tight intersections comprise of a stretching system of interfacing transmembrane proteins, for example, claudins and occludins.

The loss of epithelial obstruction uprightness and, therefore, tight intersection articulation empowers bacterial translocation over the intestinal mucosa, which can start harmful foundational irritation after extreme wounds.

Coimbra et al. demonstrated that there is expanded intestinal porousness after haemorrhagic stun and a horrendous cerebrum and consume wounds, described by a diminished tight intersection articulation.

Pharmacological, wholesome, and electrical incitement of the vagus nerve averts the breakdown of the epithelial obstruction through the adjustment of tight intersection articulation.

Proof proposes that VNS keeps up the epithelial hindrance respectability after severe damage by enteric glia actuation. A few gatherings have demonstrated that the enactment of glial cells prompts the arrival of S-nitrosoglutathione (GSNO), which expands the outflow of tight intersections and improves mucosal honesty.

These perceptions were affirmed in vivo by intraperitoneal (i.p.) infusion of GNSO in provocative models.

Vagus Nerve as well as Intestinal Immune System: The Cholinergic Anti-Inflammatory Pathway (CAIP)

For a long time, it's known that a complex interchange exists between the sensory system and resistant cells.

The focal sensory system (CNS) gets real data about the nearness of irritation and reacts appropriately employing two clear pathways: neuroendocrine and neural courses.

The afferent curve of CAIP considering unmistakable contamination, roundabout cytokines (for example, IL-1 and TNF-α) or pathogenic segments can be recognized by higher cerebrum structures circumventricular organs [CVO]) that are without a blood mind obstruction.

To be sure, the organization of intravenous (IV) endotoxin inspired c-Fos initiation in the CVO and NTS.

These structures give a direct contribution to engine neurons in the DMV, which venture vagal efferents to the spleen. Along these lines, the vagus nerve can balance the splenic invulnerable reaction.

The insusceptible framework doesn't just speak with the mind employing the flow.

On account of increasingly limited fringe irritation, in which the measure of proinflammatory cytokines isn't discernible by the CVO, afferent vagal fibers and adjoining cytokines/chemokines actuate glomus cells.

For example, IL-1 and pole cells middle people. Electrophysiological considers have announced that pole cell go-betweens and IL-1 initiate afferent vagal fibers.

Besides, both IV and IP organization of endotoxin incited c-Fos action in essential afferent ganglia (for example, nodose ganglia) trailed by expanded NTS and splenic action.

A similar c-Fos enlistment was seen in the NTS in light of intestinal hypersensitivity and aggravation brought about by careful control of the gut. Subdiaphragmatic vagotomy, to a great extent, annuls c-Fos movement in NTS and DMV after i.p. Infusion of endotoxin (for example, LPS and SEB).

Together, these perceptions unequivocally show that the mind can balance the splenic safe reaction in a roundabout way employing the location of circling cytokines and legitimately employing afferent contribution from tangible fibers.

The efferent curve of CAIP The splenic safe reaction assumes a significant job during major irritation since splenic macrophages are the substantial wellspring in TNF-α in sepsis.

In this way, the spleen is viewed as the ideal objective to regulate the insusceptible reaction in light of endotoxemia. Considering this, Borovikova et al. demonstrated that vagus nerve incitement (VNS) unequivocally restrains splenic TNF-α creation in a model of foundational aggravation, presenting the idea of the mitigating cholinergic pathway (CAIP).

This mitigating reaction is intervened by the decreased enactment of splenic macrophages communicating alpha7 nicotinic receptor (α7nAChR).

Acetylcholine (ACh) discharged by memory T cells, to be specific, interfaces with α7nAChR and hinders the emission of provocative professional cytokines through the JAK-STAT pathway.

Throughout the years, numerous investigations have demonstrated the beneficial impact of VNS in other incendiary models, for example, haemorrhagic stun, pancreatitis and collagen-incited joint pain.

We, as well as other people, likewise stretched out the idea of CAIP to the GI tract, since the gut is, to a great extent, innervated by the vagus nerve. In fact, we and others indicated that electrical nourishing and pharmacological enactment of the vagal pathway forestalls careful actuated aggravation and in this manner postoperative ileus (POI).

CAIP enactment likewise diminished intestinal aggravation in different models: diabetic-prompted gastroparesis, colitis, and LPS-incited septic ileus. Conversely, vagotomised mice have a higher defenselessness to create colitis after dextran sulfate sodium (DSS) organization.

Additionally, progressively severe colitis is likewise associated with a decrease of mucosal degrees of ACh in a model of despair.

Like in the spleen, the mitigating reaction of CAIP has interceded through *α7nAChR* macrophages.

Lack of *α7nAChR* in bone marrow-determined cells altogether repealed the vagal calming impact, while α7nAChR insufficiency in neurons and different cells didn't have a critical effect on POI, showing that the significant impact of VNS relies upon α7nAChR articulation on resistant cells instead of on neuronal cells.

As in the spleen, the CAIP isn't interceded by a direct association between *α7nAChR* macrophages and efferent vagal fibers, yet instead employing the tweak of enteric cholinergic neurons in the nearness of intestinal α7nAChR communicating macrophages.

Other mucosal and submucosal safe cells, for example, dendritic cells, pole cells, and T and B lymphocytes additionally express nicotinic receptors and may consequently be associated with CAIP.

Tachycardia

A vagal move is a move you make when you have to stop an unusually quick pulse. "Vagal" alludes to the vagus nerve. It's a long nerve that runs starting from the brain through the chest and into the stomach area.

The vagus nerve has a few capacities, including easing back the heart pulse.

There are a few basic vagal maneuvers you can do to trigger the vagus nerve to hinder a quickening pulse. This is a condition known as tachycardia.

The heart contains two regular pacemakers called the atrioventricular (AV) hub and the sinoatrial (SA) hub. The hubs are little bits of muscle tissue that help control the progression of electrical vitality through the heart.

Issues with the AV hub are at the foundation of a condition called supraventricular tachycardia (SVT). SVT is an example of quick pulses that start in the heart's upper chambers, called the atria.

At the point when the SA hub turns out to be excessively invigorated, you can encounter sinus tachycardia. This is a condition like SVT. Vagal maneuvers can be useful for sinus tachycardia as well.

Vagal maneuvers work by influencing the body's autonomic sensory system. This piece of your sensory system controls the capacities you don't need to consider, for example, pulse, absorption, respiratory rate, and others.

On account of tachycardia, a vagal maneuver can make the autonomic sensory system moderate electrical conduction through the AV hub.

The objective of a vagal maneuver is to upset the progression of electrical vitality through the heart. This permits your pulse to come back to ordinary.

There are a wide variety of types of vagal maneuvers. Every one requires your autonomic sensory system to react, basically stunning it once again into working appropriately.

Vagal maneuvers aren't consistently powerful. For individuals with genuine pulse issues, prescriptions or methods might be expected to address the tachycardia.

You may have more accomplishments with one kind of maneuver versus another. One conventional technique is the Valsalva maneuver. It takes two structures.

In one structure, essentially squeeze your nose shut and close your mouth. At that point, attempt to breathe out commandingly for around 20 seconds.

This builds circulatory strain inside the chest and powers more blood out of the chest and down the arms.

As your circulatory strain expands, the corridors and veins fix. Less blood can come back to the heart through the limited veins. That implies less blood can be siphoned out through restricted arteries. Your circulatory strain will, at that point, begin to fall.

A diminishing in pulse implies less blood can come back to the heart until you unwind and begin to inhale regularly. At the point when you do, blood will start to top off the heart.

But since your supply routes are as yet choked, less blood can leave the heart, and your pulse will rise once more. Accordingly, your pulse should begin to back off and come back to ordinary.

The other type of a Valhalla maneuver delivers a comparable response in the body. It additionally begins by holding your breath. While keeping your breath, hunker down as if you had a stable discharge. Attempt to prevent this situation for 20 seconds.

Other vagal maneuvers incorporate hacking or dunking your face in a bowl of super cold water.

Vagal maneuvers should possibly be done on the off chance that you have no different indications, for example, discombobulation, chest agony, or brevity of breath. These may be signs that you're witnessing a coronary failure.

You could be having a stroke if a quick pulse is joined by:

- an unexpected cerebral pain

- deadness on one side of the body
- loss of parity
- slurred discourse
- vision issues

Activities that reason sudden spikes in circulatory strain could cause more mischief.

There are likewise hazards related to a kind of vagal maneuver known as carotid sinus knead. It includes delicate kneading of the carotid artery. The carotid artery is situated on the privilege and left sides of the neck. From that point, it branches into two littler veins.

This move should just be finished by a specialist who knows your therapeutic history. If you have blood coagulation in your carotid artery, kneading it could send it to the cerebrum, causing a stroke.

A stable pulse rises when you exercise and afterwards returns to ordinary not long after you stop. If you have any tachycardia, physical action could trigger a quick irregular pulse that won't back off when you quit moving.

You may likewise feel your heart hustling regardless of whether you've been sitting discreetly.

If these sorts of scenes happen, hang tight for thirty minutes before you see a specialist. In any case, possibly pause if you have no different side effects or haven't got an analysis of coronary illness.

Some of the time, a scene of tachycardia will end without anyone else. Some of the time, a vagal maneuver will carry out the responsibility.

If your pulse is still high following 30 minutes, look for restorative consideration. On the off chance that your pulse quickly increments and you have different indications —, for example, chest agony, wooziness, or brevity of breath — call your nearby crisis administrations.

Tachycardia scenes can happen once to an individual, or they can be visited. The best way to appropriately analyze the condition is to have your pulse recorded on an electrocardiogram (EKG). Your EKG can help uncover the idea of your heart mood issue.

A few instances of tachycardia don't require any genuine therapeutic mediation. For specific individuals with a heart mood issue, the professionally prescribed medication adenosine (Adenocard) is useful alongside vagal maneuvers.

If you have SVT or sinus tachycardia, make sure to examine with your PCP whether vagal maneuvers are ok for you. On the off chance that they are, figure out how to do them effectively and what to do if your pulse doesn't return a short time later.

VAGUS NERVE STIMULATION (VNS)

Vagus nerve incitement is a medicinal treatment that is routinely utilized in the treatment of epilepsy and other neurological conditions. VNS contemplates clinically, yet besides logically useful concerning the job of the vagus nerve in wellbeing and ailment.

Gadget and Method

Vagus nerve incitement works by applying electrical driving forces to the vagus nerve.

The incitement of the vagus nerve can be performed in two unique manners: a direct obtrusive incitement, which is presently the most regular application, and an aberrant transcutaneous non-intrusive incitement.

Obtrusive VNS (iVNS) requires the careful implantation of a little heartbeat generator subcutaneously in the left thoracic locale.

Anodes are appended to one side cervical vagus nerve and are associated with the heartbeat generator by a lead, which is burrowed under the skin.

The generator conveys irregular electrical driving forces through the vagus nerve to the cerebrum.

It is hypothesized that these electrical motivations apply antiepileptic, stimulant, and mitigating impacts by adjusting the volatility of nerve cells. Rather than iVNS, transcutaneous VNS (tVNS) takes into account a non-obtrusive incitement of the vagus nerve with no surgery.

Here, the trigger is typically appended to the auricular concha through ear clasps and conveys electrical motivations at the subcutaneous course of the afferent auricular part of the vagus nerve.

A pilot study that inspected the utilization of VNS in 60 patients with treatment-safe burdensome issues demonstrated a noteworthy clinical improvement in 30–37% of patients and great decency.

After five years, the incitement of the vagus nerve for the treatment of recalcitrant wretchedness was endorsed by the U.S.

Nourishment and Drug Administration (FDA). From that point forward, the wellbeing and viability of VNS in gloom has been demonstrated in various observational investigations, as can be seen beneath.

Interestingly, there is no randomized, fake treatment control clinical preliminary that dependably demonstrates energizer impacts of VNS.

VNS Therapy

VNS Therapy (likewise called vagus nerve incitement) has been endorsed by the U.S. Nourishment and Drug Administration (FDA) as a new therapy for grown-ups and kids four years and more seasoned.

It is endorsed to treat focal or incomplete seizures that don't react to seizure prescriptions. This is called medicate safe epilepsy or hard-headed epilepsy.

Vagus nerve incitement (VNS) may avoid or decrease seizures by sending standard, gentle beats of electrical vitality to the cerebrum employing the vagus nerve.

The treatment comprises of a gadget that is embedded under the skin in the left chest zone. A terminal or wire is connected to the generator gadget and put under the skin. The cord is appended or twisted around the vagus nerve in the neck.

- The gadget is customized in the outpatient center to convey heartbeats or incitement at customary interims. An individual doesn't have to do anything for this gadget to work.
- An individual with a VNS gadget is typically not mindful of the incitement while it is working.
- If an individual knows about when a seizure occurs, they can swipe a magnet over the generator in the left chest territory to send an additional explosion of incitement to the cerebrum. For specific individuals, this may help stop seizures.

Vagus nerve incitement (VNS) is a kind of neuromodulation. It is intended to change how synapses work by giving electrical incitement to specific territories associated with seizures.

The vagus nerve is a piece of the autonomic sensory system, which controls elements of the body that are not under deliberate control, (for example, pulse and relaxing). The vagus nerve sends data from the cerebrum to different territories of the body. It likewise conveys data from the body to the cerebrum.

We don't know precisely how VNS functions. Research has demonstrated that VNS may help control seizures by

- Increasing bloodstream in key mind territories
- Raising levels of some mind substances (called synapses) imperative to control seizures
- Changing EEG (electroencephalogram) designs during a seizure
- 8 out of 10 individuals with epilepsy may have an expansion in their pulse before a seizure.
- In the more up to date VNS models (AspireSR and SenTivaTM), a quick increment in pulse can be gotten. This triggers a new eruption of incitement to help stop these seizures.
- These models might be particularly useful for individuals who don't know about when seizures occur, if seizures are not seen, or if seizures happen around evening time.

This treatment doesn't fix epilepsy. It's intended to help control seizures by diminishing the number and seriousness of seizures.

At first, individuals with VNS had a usual reduction in seizures by 28% in the initial three months.

A survey of 65 individuals, who had VNS for a long time or more, indicated upgrades in seizure power after some time. Seizures diminished by 36% following a half year, 58% following four years, and 75% by ten years after the VNS was put.

Different ways VNS may help individuals were accounted for in an investigation of 112 grown-ups with focal epilepsy that didn't react to medications.

Individuals were set in two groups:

1. VNS treatment and best therapeutic practice
2. No VNS yet got best medicinal practice. Data was gathered over one year. Consequences of this examination appeared:

Recuperation time after a seizure might be shorter for specific individuals.

8 of 10 individuals revealed an improved personal satisfaction.

Around 6 of 10 detailed less stress over seizures and improved sharpness.

A large portion of the individuals announced that their seizures were less acute.

VNS is utilized for individuals with refractory or tranquilize safe epilepsy. This implies seizures are not controlled in the wake of attempting, in any event, two appropriate seizure prescriptions.

It's a particular treatment, which implies it is utilized notwithstanding seizure prescriptions. For specific individuals, when VNS functions admirably, the portion or utilization of a seizure prescription might be diminished.

VNS is typically utilized if an individual can't have epilepsy medical procedures or if the medical system doesn't work.

Once in a while, an individual might be offered VNS if different reasons make medical procedures unrealistic.

While considering VNS, in a perfect world, an individual is first observed at a thorough epilepsy focus to ensure that the total of what alternatives have been investigated and that the system is directly for them.

VNS won't help seizures that are not epileptic and not related to electrical movement in the cerebrum.

It's mostly shown for focal seizures, yet individuals with certain sorts of summed up seizures, including Lennox Gastaut Syndrome, have improved as well.

It's imperative to check whether different variables might be influencing seizures and to treat those things first.

For instance, if an individual is experiencing difficulty taking meds consistently or has another way of life factors influencing seizures, directing and instruction about trigger administration would be required first.

An epilepsy master would audit the sorts of prescriptions that you have attempted and ensure that you have tried the right medications for the correct kind of seizures. What's more, tried them for a long enough timeframe.

Individuals with noteworthy asthma or other breathing issues, rest apnea, or some heart issues might be urged against utilizing vagus nerve incitement. In some cases, medicinal other problems like these could deteriorate with VNS.

Anybody considering VNS (or any gadget) should check first with their essential consideration specialist to ensure this is directly for them.

Individuals with just a single vagus nerve would not be a high possibility for VNS.

Individuals who have had strange heart rhythms (arrhythmias) or a low pulse (bradycardia) ought not to utilize the auto-stimulation settings in the more up to date VNS models.

The Neural Mechanism of VNS

The system by which VNS may profit patients nonresponsive to conventional antidepressants is misty, with further research expected to explain this.

Utilitarian neuroimaging ponders affirmed that VNS adjusts the movement of numerous cortical and subcortical areas.

Through immediate or circuitous anatomic associations employing the NTS, the vagus nerve has auxiliary associations with a few states of mind directing limbic and cortical cerebrum zones.

Consequently, in interminable VNS for misery, PET outputs demonstrated a decrease in resting cerebrum movement in the ventromedial prefrontal cortex (vmPFC), which activities to the amygdala and other mind locales regulating feeling.

VNS brings about synthetic changes in monoamine digestion in these locales, conceivably bringing about the upper activity. Different kinds of proof have appeared for the connection between monoamine and energizer activity.

All medications that expansion monoamines serotonin (5-HT), NE, or dopamine (DA) in the synaptic parted have stimulant properties.

In like manner, exhaustion of monoamines incites burdensome manifestations in people who have an expanded danger of discouragement.

Constant VNS impacts the centralization of 5-HT, NE, and DA in the cerebrum and the cerebrospinal liquid. In rodents, it has been demonstrated that VNS medicines incite huge time-subordinate increments in basal neuronal terminating in the brainstem cores for serotonin in the dorsal raphe nucleus.

Therefore, continuous VNS was related to expanded extracellular degrees of serotonin in the dorsal raphe.

A few lines of proof recommend that NE is a synapse critical in the pathophysiology and treatment of the complicated issue.

Therefore, trial consumption of NE in the cerebrum prompted an arrival of burdensome side effects after fruitful treatment with NE stimulant medications.

The LC contains the most significant populace of noradrenergic neurons in mind and gets projections from NTS, which, thus, receives an afferent contribution from the vagus nerve. In this manner, VNS prompts an upgrade of the terminating movement of NE neurons.

Therefore, an expansion in the terminating action of serotonin neurons. In this way, VNS was appeared to expand the NE fixation in the prefrontal cortex. The pharmacologic pulverization of noradrenergic neurons brought about the loss of upper VNS impacts.

If there should be an occurrence of DA, it has been demonstrated that the momentary impacts and the long haul impacts of VNS in the treatment of safe significant wretchedness may prompt brainstem dopaminergic initiation.

DA is a catecholamine that, to a considerable degree, is integrated into the gut and assumes an essential job in the prize framework in the cerebrum.

Further, valuable impacts of VNS may be applied through a monoamine-free way.

Along these lines, VNS medications may bring about significant changes of monoamine metabolites in the hippocampus, and a few investigations detailed the impact of VNS on hippocampal neurogenesis.

This procedure has been viewed as a critical natural procedure vital for keeping up the normal state of mind.

Serotonin is additionally a significant synapse in the gut that can animate peristalsis and instigate sickness and retching by initiating the vagus nerve.

Moreover, it is fundamental for the guideline of essential capacities, for example, craving and rest, and adds to sentiments of prosperity.

Ninety fiver percent of it is delivered by enterochromaffin cells, a kind of neuroendocrine cell that lives close by the epithelium covering the lumen of the stomach related tract.

Serotonin is discharged from enterochromaffin cells because of mechanical or substance incitement of the gastrointestinal tract, which prompts actuation of 5-HT3 receptors on the terminals of vagal afferents.

5-HT3 receptors are likewise present on the soma of vagal afferent neurons, including gastrointestinal vagal afferent neurons, where they can be actuated by flowing 5-HT.

The focal terminals of vagal afferents likewise display 5-HT3 receptors that capacity to increment glutamatergic synaptic transmission to second request neurons of the nucleus tractus solitarius inside the brainstem.

Subsequently, connections between the vagus nerve and serotonin frameworks in the gut and the mind seem to assume a significant job in the treatment of mental conditions.

YOGA

The vagus nerve assumes a focal job in your enthusiastic and physical wellbeing. The vagus nerve reaches out, starting from the brainstem into your stomach and digestive organs, enervating your heart and lungs and associating your throat and facial muscles.

Like this, any yoga rehearses that invigorate these regions of the body can impact the tone of the vagus nerve. Vagus nerve yoga encourages you to recover equalization of body and mind utilizing devices of care, mindful breathing, and physical stances.

Your sensory system is worked around the equalization of two restricting activities.

The thoughtful sensory system is related to the battle or flight reaction that is the aftereffect of the arrival of cortisol (synthetic stress concoctions) all through the circulatory system. The parasympathetic is related to unwinding, absorption, and recovery.

These two pieces of your autonomic sensory system are intended to work in musical shift, a procedure that supports sound rhythms of sharpness and peacefulness that encourage physical and emotional wellness.

Shockingly, constant pressure and uncertain injury meddle with the harmony between the reflective and parasympathetic elements of your sensory system.

Since we experience a day to day reality such that is over-invigorating and enacting for the thoughtful sensory system, a significant number of us need access to apparatuses that assist us with engaging the parasympathetic sensory system consistently.

The vagus nerve has an inhibitory impact on the thoughtful sensory system action. Rehearses that invigorate the vagus nerve has a quieting effect on your body and brain.

It is likewise imperative to perceive that people with uncertain PTSD frequently resort to a crude articulation of the parasympathetic sensory system, which can prompt side effects of weakness or discouragement.

At the point when left untreated, ceaseless pressure and uncertain PTSD can upset your physical, mental, and enthusiastic wellbeing.

Fortunately rehearses that emphasis on invigorating the vagus nerve can help recapture balance if you are either keyed-up with uneasiness or shut down with weariness.

An expansion in vagal tone is connected to a decrease in irritation and better anticipation in individuals experiencing ceaseless disease, nervousness, or discouragement.

Vagal tone is estimated in the adjustments in a pulse that happen with the breath. This is alluded to as Heart pulse Variability or HRV. Solid vagal tone includes a slight increment in pulse on the inward breath and a diminishing of the pulse when you breathe out.

Vagal tone can be seen as an ideal balance of the negative and neutral behavior of the rest of the body.

Individuals with higher HRV could move all the more effectively from energy to lose and can recuperate all the more effectively from stress.

You can figure out how to direct the working of your vagus nerve with procedures, for example, adjusting the cadence of your breath, rehearsing careful body mindfulness, and investigating physical yoga stances to make a more prominent decision about your degree of excitement or initiation. For instance, with substantial mindfulness, you can adjust your breathing mood to encourage a condition of loosened up sharpness.

This can assist you with taking advantage of an ideal degree of center and consideration that is frequently depicted as a being in the zone or the experience of the stream that powers your innovativeness. Likewise, you can learn explicit breath rehearses that assist you with unwinding at night and plan for tranquil rest.

The objective of a vagus nerve yoga practice is to turn out to be progressively adaptable, not of the physical body yet of the sensory system. Research has indicated huge advantages of yoga for expanded vagal tone, stress decrease, and injury recuperation.

This will assist you with getting gifted at exchanging among thoughtful and parasympathetic sensory systems without hardly lifting a finger and decision. The accompanying seven vagus nerve yoga practices will help you with creating sound vagal tone, invigorate as required, unwind as wanted, and recover balance in your life:

- **Conscious Breathing**: The quickest approach to change the equalization of thoughtful and parasympathetic sensory system activities is with the breath.

To offset any over-stimulation of the thoughtful sensory system, vagus nerve yoga centers on diaphragmatic breathing and broadening the length of the breath out.

Research has discovered that moderate, cadenced, diaphragmatic breathing builds solid vagal tone. One type of yogic breathing is *Ujjayi pranayama,* which makes a slight narrowing in the rear of the throat by engaging your murmur muscles.

To get familiar with this breath, breathe out of your mouth as though you are misting up a mirror. Presently, breathe similarly yet close your mouth and breathe out of your nose.

You will see the sound of your breath is stronger, which regularly seems like the floods of the sea. Start evenly, means you're breathing in and breathing out. For significantly more profound unwinding, step by step increments the length of your breathing out when contrasted with the breathe-in.

For instance, you may begin with a 4-round on the breathing in and breathe out, the breath out to a 6 or 8 tally. This has a quieting impact on your parasympathetic sensory system.

- **Half-Smile**: Engaging a "half-grin" is a significant method to change your psychological state and develop a tranquil inclination at the time.

Since the vagus nerve stretches out into the muscles of the face, you can increment vagal tone by loosening up the muscles of your face and afterwards marginally turning up your lips. This training engages what Dr. Stephen Porges calls the "social sensory system," the most developed part of the vagus nerve.

As you grin, envision your jaw mellowing and a casual inclination spreading over your face, your whole head, and down your shoulders. Notice the simple changes like your musings and feelings.

- **Open your Heart**: You can tenderly animate the vagus nerve with yoga poses that open over your chest and throat.

Attempt this delicate situated heart-opening practice by carrying your hands to your shoulders. Breathe in as you extend over the front of your chest, open your elbows wide, and lift your jaw.

Breathe out as you contract your elbows before your heart and fold your jawline. Take a few full breaths in this moving reflection.

Concentrating on your inward breath in this breath example can be invigorating and elevating. Enable yourself to venture away from any confining influence heart.

- memories getting up in the first part of the day or the event that you are feeling worn out and weary toward the evening, yoga can give a delicate jolt of energy for your brain and body.

Investigate standing stances such as warrior (virabhadrasana) posture to invigorate your brain and wake up your body. Notice the association of your feet to the earth remains grounded to empower yourself reasonably.

Enable the breath to stay cadenced with the goal that you visit attached and associated with the sensations in your body

- **Release the Belly**: You can work with the association of the vagus nerve as it goes through your gut. Discover your way into a table situation with your hands underneath your shoulders and your knees underneath your hips. If there is any inconvenience on your knees, you can put a collapsed cover underneath you. As you breathe in, lift your head and your hips, bringing down your midsection towards the floor as you move into Cow Pose.

On your breathing out lower your head and hips while you lift your spine into a Cat Pose.

Locate your very own planning of the development with your breath. Rehash the same amount of times as you like making a delicate back rub for your midsection and spine.

- **Self-Compassion or "Cherishing Kindness" Meditation:**

Self-empathy and the act of "adoring thoughtfulness" request that you engage in the demonstration of friendship toward yourself as well as other people.

Research on that person who practices a caring generosity contemplation uncovered expanded vagal tone, more prominent autonomic adaptability, a developed feeling of social connectedness, and increasingly constructive feelings.

Pause for a minute to consider a test you are looking in your life. Presently, envision another person confronting a comparable analysis.

Would you be able to bring out a feeling of empathy or benevolence toward this other individual? Notice how this sentiment of sympathy feels in your body. Wish them well.

Check whether you would be able to expand that similar nature of adoring generosity toward yourself? Wish yourself well.

- **Yoga Nidra**: Restorative yoga can assist you with backing off and quiet the sensory system. One exemplary practice is Yoga Nidra, which is frequently alluded to as "yogic rest" or a reflection in unwinding.

Yoga Nidra is the cure to our unpleasant, current way of life and offers a chance to reestablish body and psyche through getting to the parasympathetic sensory system. When you locate a loosening up position lying on the floor, cover, or yoga tangle, develop attention to your body and breathe.

Make space for anything that you are feeling, including any regions of pressure, largeness, or tightening. Enable yourself to stay still for 30 minutes for a profoundly unwinding and supporting experience.

When exposed to Cold

Direct stimulation of the vagus nerve is just conceivable with the assistance of an embedded gadget that produces electric heartbeats.

Be that as it may, because the vagus nerve is associated with numerous pieces of your body, invigorating certain territories of your body will have a backhanded positive effect on vagal tone, as the body reroutes this stimulation back to the vagus nerve.

Beneath, we will clarify some healthy ways to, in a roundabout way, invigorate the vagus nerve.

Presenting your body to intense virus conditions, for example, scrubbing down or sprinkling cold water all over, builds stimulation of the vagus nerve. While your body acclimates to the chilly, thoughtful movement decays, while parasympathetic action increments.

It has been seen that presentation to cold actuates the vagus nerve since it invigorates the cholinergic neurons crossing these innervations. An examination led at the University of Oulu has uncovered that ordinary introduction to cold decreases the battle flight reaction that dispatches the thoughtful sensory system.

It tends to be sufficient for a virus shower of 30 seconds per day or a virus towel on the face. There are additionally the individuals who rest on the tummy, putting a 3D shape of ice on the scruff. Others like to drink a glass of cold water rapidly.

Breathing

You can, by implication, manipulate the vagus nerve by taking deep, deliberate breaths from your stomach. Profound breathing enacts explicit neurons that identify the circulatory strain.

These neurons sign to the vagus nerve that circulatory strain is getting excessively high, and the vagus nerve thus reacts by bringing down your pulse.

A great many people breathe in the air somewhere in the range of 10 and 14 times each moment, which implies they have a shallow relaxing.

The perfect is to breathe in the air six times each moment. This way, another hugely successful vagal stimulation method comprises breathing profoundly.

The diaphragmatic taking specifically enacts the vagus nerve, and the cerebrum translates it as it is essential to quiet down, regardless of whether the nerve has not given that request explicitly.

The instrument is the equivalent for which, if you close your eyes and make taps with your fingers on your eyelids, you will see short flashes of light because the cerebrum deciphers them so.

With diaphragmatic breathing, we make more profound breathing that carries air into the lower some portion of the chest, utilizing the stomach effectively and advancing unwinding.

Effects on Mental and Physical Health

Although the vagus nerve influences organs outside of the focal sensory system, or CNS, which comprises of the mind and spinal line, recall that the vagus nerve is established in the brainstem and cerebellum.

Ideal vagus nerve capacity, or "high vagal tone list," is related to robust social associations, positive feelings, and better physical wellbeing. People with low vagal tone list experience sadness, coronary episodes, depression, adverse sentiments, and stroke.

Mind wellbeing and gut wellbeing impact each other, and the vagus nerve is correctly the connection between the two. The vagal tone list can be thought of as the body's "gut feeling" that gets passed on straightforwardly to the mind and creates a criticism circle of more fabulous inspiration or greater antagonism.

Rising examinations show that the vagal tone record is dictated by signals discharged from the invulnerable framework called cytokines.

Research is in progress to all the more likely see how refreshing the vagus nerve offers the potential for treating incendiary conditions, for example, rheumatoid joint inflammation, without the utilization of pharmaceutical medications.

VAGUS NERVE STIMULATION (CONTINUED)

Benefits of Vagus Nerve Stimulation

Vagus nerve brokenness results typically from a low vagal tone record, so stimulating the vagus nerve can operate as a heal for the signs, manifestations, and infections recorded previously.

A large number of these types of treatment speak to the way of life changes meaning. It is sheltered to embrace more than one of the accompanying practices to expand the vagal tone file.

Add fish to the eating regimen

The EPA and DHA found in fish animate the vagus nerve to build pulse inconstancy and lower pulse. These impacts can be obtained from a fish oil supplement also.

Become a yogi

Yoga supports the state of mind and brings down tension as well as expands vagus nerve and parasympathetic framework action. The moderate, profound breathing-related benefits of yoga enact exceptionally delicate weight receptors in the heart and neck called baroreceptors, which send a sign to the mind telling it to initiate the vagus nerve.

Form social associations

Research shows social connections make people feel nearer to other people, and that feeling invigorates the vagus nerve.

Generously chew gum

Biting gum supports the arrival of the hormone, CCK, from the gut, which encourages correspondence from the vagus nerve to the mind.

Hack or agreement the stomach muscles

The sensation felt while hacking or having a stable discharge is created by the vagus nerve, so reenacting these exercises animates the vagus nerve.

Eat more fiber

Fiber builds GLP-1, a hormone that supports correspondence between the vagus nerve and cerebrum, and eases back stomach exhausting and makes the body feel full more.

Engage the larynx

Exercises like singing, rinsing, or in any event, initiating the gag reflex, engage the larynx in this manner invigorating the vagus nerve. For help with enacting the gag reflex, utilize a tongue depressor or spoon.

Exercise routinely

Exercise animates the vagus nerve to invigorate gut stream, subsequently profiting the vagal file alongside discharge.

Fast irregularly

Irregular fasting decreases the number of calories expended. That decrease in calories causes pulse changeability to spike and digestion to dive—two occasions that trigger vagus nerve work.

Discover an acupuncturist

Conventional needle therapy, particularly to the ear, invigorates the vagus nerve.

Get immediate daylight

UVA beams increment the body's degrees of melanocyte animating hormone (MSH), another hormone that invigorates the vagus nerve. UVB beams increment the quantity of MSH receptors all through the body, making it workable for considerably more MSH to tie.

Incorporate petition each day

Studies show asking invigorates the vagus nerve by expanding diastolic circulatory strain and pulse fluctuation. These impacts generally upgrade cardiovascular wellbeing.

Giggle regularly

Yeah, Lol. The association among giggling and the vagal tone was first found because of individuals blacking out from occasions that include the body hunkering down, for example, hacking, snickering, moving the guts, gulping, and peeing. The blacking out comes from different disorders, including the vagus nerve; however, in reliable people, chuckling bolsters better insight while avoiding coronary illness.

Figure out how to adore cold temperatures

Acclimating to temperatures colder than average internal heat level triggers the PNS enthusiastically employing vagus nerve Stimulation. This impact is best accomplished by drinking cold water, dunking the face in freshwater, or scrubbing down.

Think every day

Thinking to advance love and generosity inside the soul builds the vagal tone list. Om reciting is an elective technique for contemplation that delivers a similar impact.

Practice Tai Chi

Studies show Tai Chi builds pulse changeability, demonstrating it accomplishes this by enacting the vagus nerve.

Have kneaded regularly

Neck and foot rubs animate the Vagus Nerve while lessening the danger of seizures and coronary illness, separately. Entire body pressure rubs animate gut work, which in a roundabout way actuates the vagus nerve.

Rest on the correct side

Lying on the back diminishes vagus nerve enactment, yet resting on the right side shows more noteworthy Vagus Nerve stimulation contrasted with left side dozing.

Invest some energy with Nervana

Nervana is a type of innovation intended to animate the vagus nerve through electrical waves matched up with music. Accessible as an uneven generator or double-sided earphones, Nervana triggers synapse discharge from the cerebrum and instigates quiet inside the psyche and body.

Supplement zinc and serotonin (5-HTP)

Zinc is critical to vagus nerve work, and numerous individuals accidentally lack this mineral. Serotonin enacts the vagus nerve through a few distinct receptors in the body.

Take a probioticOptimising gut wellbeing is perfect for boosting Vagus Nerve Stimulation. Taking a probiotic can guarantee this, particularly the probiotic, Lactobacillus rhamnosus, which improved the capacity of GABA receptors for the vagus nerve in creature considers.

Attempt a douche

Speeding up the development of the entrails grows the digestive organs and actuates vagus nerve movement.

Utilize Pulsed Electromagnetic Field (PEMF) treatment

Research affirms that attractive fields animate the vagus nerve by expanding pulse inconstancy. Utilizing a gadget that invigorates beat beautiful field waves straightforwardly on the gut, head, and neck will focus on the vagus nerve.

Work the vocal harmonies

Reciting, murmuring, singing, talking, and other vocal harmony practices increment pulse fluctuation, which initiates the vagus nerve.

A Germaine Note on Gluten and the Vagus Nerve

People delicate to gluten can encounter irritation and cerebrum issue, including nervousness, mental imbalance, ADHD, bipolar issue, gloom, schizophrenia, Alzheimer's malady, or Parkinson's sickness.

Such gluten affectability likewise upsets gut wellbeing bringing about a decreased vagal list. Along these lines, stopping the utilization of gluten is one more approach to invigorate the vagus nerve while supporting gut wellbeing and diminishing irritation in mind.

Studies show vagus nerve stimulation additionally brings down circulatory strain, diminishes pulse, decreases the body's reaction to push, and improves absorption.

Past without gluten Foods

Expending a sans gluten diet goes past looking for without gluten nourishments. The perfect without gluten diet incorporates cell reinforcement rich nourishments and different nourishments wealthy in ubiquinone and acetyl-L-carnitine, which shield the cerebrum from oxidative harm.

An Integrative Health Practitioner can give some astounding dietary choices to keeping up a without gluten diet.

Instigated significant changes in mind bloodstream Positron-outflow tomography and functional, attractive reverberation imaging of the impacts of VNS in individuals have affirmed the impact the vagus nerve on higher cerebrum structures.

Stimulation of VNS causes increments in the cerebral bloodstream and can change electroencephalographic examples. Clinical examinations with positron-outflow tomography demonstrated that VNS expanded the bloodstream to the right thalamus.

The correct back fleeting cortex, the left putamen, and the left substandard cerebellum at interictal phase of seizures; Clinical investigations with useful, attractive reverberation imaging showed that the territories of critical actuation in light of VNS were the two-sided orbitofrontal and parietooccipital cortex, the left transient cortex, and the left amygdala at interictal phase of seizures.

Creature study demonstrated that VNS could arrest ongoing seizure movement (ictal phase of seizures) by eventually diminishing the hippocampal bloodstream.

Against neuroinflammation or immunomodulation

Full trial and clinical proof backings a connection among aggravation and epilepsy, both as far as epileptogenesis and the long haul outcomes of seizures, which shows that initiation of provocative procedures in mind is a typical component of the different epileptic issue.

With a flawless vagal-invulnerable system, VNS can hose a provocative reaction.

The vagus nerve is trapped in immunome as efferent vagus nerve fibers foundationally hinder parahippocampal diminishes in glucose digestion and bloodstream, immunomodulation, or against neuroinflammation.

Change EEG cerebrum practical availability just as adjustment of neuronal movement and the proteome of excitatory neurotransmitters of amygdaloid piriform cortex, and conceivable tweak of adenosine framework and DNA methylation.

Comorbidities in epilepsy speak to a significant applied and remedial test.

Right now, the bidirectional connection among epilepsy and related comorbidities has been paid an ever-increasing number of considerations, and advances on the cover of mental subjective and neurologic side effects from a pathophysiologic and phenomenological point of view are turning into a hotly debated issue in epilepsy.

The problematic issue is the most widely recognized kind of mental comorbidity in patients with epilepsy, particularly in people experiencing unmanageable fleeting projection epilepsy.

A few instruments of essential burdensome issue, for example, endocrine variations from the norm, auxiliary and practical irregularities of cortical and subcortical structures, synapse anomalies, and immunological aggravation variations from the norm, affect cortical hyperexcitability and the epileptogenic procedure.

The component of VNS to treat epilepsy-related comorbidities may be through the systems referenced above. Of logical intriguing, movement in VNS clinical viability after some time and ceaseless.

VNS actuates permanent changes in the neuronal system engaged with epileptogenesis, showing that extended haul utilization of VNS adjusts the movement of epilepsy (sickness alteration or antiepileptogenesis) and that the previous this is done, the better the result for seizures and related comorbidities control.

In this piece, we will concentrate on the methods of activity of VNS for epilepsy and related comorbidities.

Methods of Action of VNS for Epilepsy

Serotonin as a middle man of the antiepileptic impacts of VNS. The ongoing investigation gave persuading proof to the presence of a stable causal connection between expanded noradrenergic flagging and the anticonvulsant effect of VNS.

Expanded in extracellular hippocampal noradrenaline (NE), however, not of dopamine, serotonin and GABA is liable for it.

What's more, VNS actuates the hypothalamic-pituitary-adrenal hub. Creature explore has demonstrated that VNS-actuated expanded hippocampal articulation of corticotrophin discharging factor and expanded plasma levels of adrenocorticotropic hormone and corticosterone, which bolster the job of the VNS in immunomodulation or hostile to neuroinflammation.

Change EEG mind useful availability EEG cerebrum utilitarian network is an approach to ponder cerebrum work through the investigation of pairwise connections and reflects how different mind territories arrange their exercises.

Evaluating changes of EEG mind useful availability is shown as a promising instrument for anticipating reaction to VNS.

The impact of VNS on utilitarian availability has been contemplated utilizing scalp EEG demonstrated that useful network would, in general, be lower in the on period and that this impact was maximal for responder understanding.

All the more as of late, the study explored the effect of VNS on the minded useful network with stereotactic EEG signals. The outcomes demonstrated that VNS could diminish or expand the beneficial availability changes with variable impact from patient to tolerant, and clinical responder with the diminished useful network.

Change the proteome of excitatory neural connections of amygdaloid/piriform cortex.

The atomic systems basic VNS for epilepsy are in general misty. The versatility of excitatory neural connections is thought to add to the hyperexcitability of epilepsy.

The postsynaptic thickness (PSD) is a layer specialization of the postsynaptic segment of excitatory neurotransmitters in the CNS, and the protein organization of the PSD is directed by neuronal movement.

The ongoing examination demonstrated that VNS adjusts both neuronal movement in the amygdala and hippocampus and the arrangement of excitatory neurotransmitters in the CNS, which recommended that subordinate action development of excitatory neurotransmitters may be atomic focuses of VNS for epilepsy.

Regulation of adenosine framework and DNA methylation Adenosine is an inhibitory modulator of cerebrum action, and its anticonvulsant and seizure ending impacts, interceded by both receptor-ward and receptor-free pathways, have been illustrated in a full scope of experimental models of epilepsy and clinical investigations.

Helpful adenosine growth is a fantastic therapeutic strategy to stifle epileptic seizures and epileptogenesis.

Neuro-stimulation has been shown to expand the extracellular adenosine fixation in the cerebrum to upgrade adenosine flagging and adenosine A1 receptor-subordinate actuation.

Then again, the increment of adenosine levels in the cerebrum may likewise apply receptor-free impacts in DNA methylation homeostasis to decrease DNA methylation.

There is each sign that operators ready to expand adenosine accessibility may have a spot later on the treatment of epilepsy employing adenosine receptor-subordinate pathway and adenosine receptor-free pathway.

How the VNS adjusted adenosine framework and exerted its adequacy in the treatment of epilepsy and alteration, the movement of epilepsy needs further examination later on.

Instruments of activity of VNS for comorbidities related to epilepsy

Epilepsy is a turmoil of the cerebrum describe by a suffering inclination to generate epileptic seizures and by the neurobiological, intellectual, mental, and social results of this condition.

Around 30 percent of patients with epilepsy is pharmacoresistant and separated from the individuals who are a contender for a particular medical procedure; most will keep on having handicapping seizures and the low quality of existence with a full scope of subjective and mental side effects.

Repetitive seizures incited the rearrangement of neural circuits and exercises in the cerebrum; along these lines, patients, much of the time, experience subjective, mental and temperament issues.

Then again, the latest research shows that some neurocognitive and mental comorbidities just as auxiliary cerebrum changes originate before the beginning of seizures, with the new psychological trade-off being additionally amplified by the beginning of epileptogenesis, and later on, by the chronicity of seizures.

Epilepsy, being viewed as a model of neuropsychiatric neurocognitive and ailment, and related comorbidities, usually are successive and share regular fundamental components with epilepsy.

As of now, the bidirectional connection among epilepsy and related comorbidities has been paid significantly more considerations.

Neuropsychiatry

As of now, components of dysregulation of the nerve centre pituitary–adrenal (HPA) pivot, and traded off raphe-hippocampal serotonergic transmission are very much acknowledged behind epilepsy and neuropsychiatric issue.

VNS has been demonstrated to expand the basal terminating rates of serotonergic neurons in the dorsal raphe nucleus, in this way, assumes a job in the two seizures and related comorbidities.

As of late, adenosine brokenness has been shown as the hidden instrument for comorbidities related to epilepsy and that significant adenosine expansion may be compelling for the treatment of epilepsy and comorbid side effects in epilepsy.

Clinical just as preliminary information propose that a set of three of synaptotoxicity, astrogliosis, and overexpression of ADK, bringing about the insufficiency of homeostatic adenosine can straightforwardly cause a full scope of psychological and mental indications ordinarily observed as comorbidities in epilepsy as pursues:

Adenosine and epilepsy

As presented above, ample experimental and clinical proof demonstrated that useless astrocytic adenosine homeostasis as one of the early pathophysiologic systems of epilepsy, and significant adenosine expansion applies anticonvulsant and seizure ending impacts, intervened by both receptorward and receptor–autonomous pathways.

Adenosine and comprehension

Adenosine influences subjective procedures on a few unthinking levels through privately refined neuronal and astroglial A2AR flagging impacts and adjustment of glutamatergic, dopaminergic, GABAergic, and BDNF-subordinate components.

Cancellation of adenosine A2A receptors from astrocytes disturbs glutamate homeostasis, promoting psychological weakness. Adenosine enlargement to the hippocampus can improve work.

These discoveries recommend that significant adenosine expansion may comprise a promising methodology for the treatment of comorbid discouragement in a full scope of the neurological and neuropsychiatric issues.

Adenosine and also Depression

The ongoing examination demonstrated that astrocytic motioning to adenosine A1 receptor was required for the hearty decrease of burdensome like practices in mice following 12h of lack of sleep.

Approaches referred to build adenosine levels, for example, practice, lack of sleep, needle therapy, deep mind stimulation, or ketogenic diet, have demonstrated upper impacts. S-adenosylhomocysteine, a forerunner of adenosine, has been utilized for the treatment of significant grief.

VNS, the most ordinarily utilized neuromodulation for pharmacoresistant epilepsy, may establish a promising methodology for the treatment of epilepsy-related comorbidities too through adenosine framework.

Aetna

Aetna considers vagus nerve electrical triggers medicinally essential robust therapeutic hardware (DME) for shortening the term or diminishing the seriousness of seizures in individuals with focal seizures (previously known as incomplete beginning seizures).

Who stay recalcitrant to ideal anti-epileptic prescriptions as well as careful intercession, (for example, a lesionectomy or average fleeting lobectomy), or who have crippling side effects from anti-epileptic drugs, and who have no history of a two-sided or left cervical vagotomy. (Note: Electronic examination of an embedded neurostimulator beat generator framework for vagus nerve stimulation is viewed as restoratively fundamental when criteria are met).

Aetna considers vagus nerve electrical triggers restoratively essential active medicinal gear (DME) for the treatment of Lennox-Gastaut disorder in individuals who stay headstrong to ideal anti-epileptic meds, and additionally careful intercession, (for example, a corpus callosotomy or lesional epilepsy medical procedure), or who have incapacitating side effects from antiepileptic drugs, and who have no history of a respective or left cervical vagotomy.

Aetna thinks about substitution/update of a vagus nerve treatment framework/handheld magnet restoratively fundamental if the first framework/magnet met criteria as therapeutically essential and is never again under guarantee and can't be fixed.

Aetna considers transcutaneous vagus nerve stimulation experimental and investigational for the treatment of seizures and every single other sign (see beneath) because the effectiveness of this methodology has not been built up.

Aetna considers vagus nerve electrical triggers and transcutaneous vagus nerve stimulation experimental and investigational for the avoidance of incessant headache assaults because the effectiveness of this methodology has not been set up.

Aetna considers vagus nerve electrical triggers, and transcutaneous vagus nerve stimulation experimental and investigational for the treatment of every single other sign since its effectiveness for these signs have not been built up (not a comprehensive rundown though);

Addictions. Alzheimer. Sickness. Anxiety issue. Atonic seizures. Atrial fibrillation. Autism. Bipolar problem, Bulimia Nervosa, Cerebral paralysis, Crohn's ailment, Chronic migraines, Cluster migraines, Cognitive weakness related with Alzheimer's sickness, Coma, Depression, Dravet disorder, Eating issue (e.g., anorexia and bulimia), Essential tremor, Fibromyalgia, Generalized engine seizures (some time ago summed up tonic- clonic seizures), Generalized epilepsy disorders, Generalized treatment-resistant epilepsy, Heart disappointment, Hemicrania Traumatic mind damage (TBI) including post-TBI pneumonia.

Vagus nerve obstructing for being Obese.

Data

Roughly 1.7 million Americans suffer from epilepsy. Most by far of these patients can be constrained by conventional medication treatment. In spite of the accessibility of new antiepileptic drugs and advances in careful treatment, more than 200,000 individuals stay unmanageable to treatment.

Vagus nerve stimulation (VNS) utilizing the NeuroCybernetic Prosthesis (NCP) System has been appeared to abbreviate the term and lessen the seriousness of seizures in specific patients who stay unmanageable in spite of ideal medication treatment or careful intercession or in those with incapacitating side effects of antiepileptic prescriptions.

The vagus nerve sends a sign to the cerebrum, which invigorates the zone of the mind accepted to be associated with temperament guideline and seizure movement; in any case, the particular instrument of activity is obscure.

The NCP System, affirmed by the Food and Drug Administration (FDA) on July 16, 1997, is a pacer-like gadget embedded under the skin in the upper left chest territory.

It is associated by wire to a lead that is folded over the left vagus nerve in the neck. Through the vagus nerve, it conveys irregular electrical heartbeats 24 hours per day to the cerebrum.

The lead terminal stimulation is performed distinctly on the left vagal nerve, as the privilege vagal nerve helps control the heartbeat. At the point when a patient detects the approaching beginning of a seizure, he/she can enact the gadget through a hand-held magnet to convey an extra portion of stimulation.

The beat generator can be customized to convey stimulation inside parameters that suit the person's needs. Treatment with the vagus nerve trigger isn't free of side effects. Patients have encountered hack, raspiness, changes in their voice, and brevity of breath.

Late examinations have built up vagus nerve stimulation to be a practical alternative for improving seizure control in difficult to treat pediatric patients with epilepsy.

An appraisal of VNS in youngsters by the National Institute for Clinical Excellence (NICE, 2004) arrived at the accompanying resolution: "Current proof on the security and efficacy of vagus nerve stimulation for unmanageable epilepsy in kids seems sufficient to help the utilization of this methodology, given that the ordinary game plans are set up for assent, review and clinical administration."

Vagus nerve stimulation (VNS) was initially structured as a treatment alternative for therapeutically headstrong epilepsy or the failure to control seizure movement with antiepileptic tranquilize treatment.

Notwithstanding, VNS has additionally been proposed as an assistant treatment for treatment safe significant melancholy and bipolar issue. VNS is being examined for an expansive scope of signs including Alzheimer's sickness, uneasiness issue, bulimia, constant cerebral pain/headache, cardiovascular breakdown, and weight.

It has been accounted for that VNS in patients with epilepsy is related to a perking up. Around 1/3 of patients with significant severe issues neglect to encounter sufficient side effect improvement in spite of satisfactory treatment.

The executives of patients with treatment safe misery (TRD) typically comprises of pharmacological or non-pharmacological strategies.

The previous methodology involves changing to another antidepressant monotherapy, and growth or blend with at least two antidepressants or different operators.

The latter approach incorporates psychotherapy, electroconvulsive treatment, and VNS. Even though VNS is related to a state of mind upgrades in patients with epilepsy, randomized, controlled examinations with long-term follow-up are expected to affirm its effect on TRD.

In such a manner, Kosel and Schlaepfer (2003) expressed that ongoing information from an open-label, multi-centre pilot study, including 60 patients, proposed a potential clinical convenience in the intense and support treatment of TRD.

Notwithstanding, distinct restorative effects of clinical hugeness stay to be affirmed in enormous placebo-controlled preliminary.

This is in concurrence with the perception of George et al. (2000) who noticed that further research is expected to explain the instruments of activity of VNS and its potential clinical utility in the administration of patients with TRD.

Due to the absence of well-designed controlled clinical preliminaries, VNS for unmanageable melancholy is viewed as experimental and investigational.

Long-term information seeing mediocrity just as significant and practical results of discouraged patients getting VNS are expected to learn the effectiveness of this methodology for treating stubborn sadness.

An evaluation by the Institute for Clinical Systems Improvement (ICSI, 2004) expressed that VNS for despondency "can't be considered evidence-based."

In an intense stage pilot study (n = 59), Nahas et al. (2005) assessed the wellbeing and effectiveness of VNS for patients with the treatment-resistant significant burdensome scene (MDE).

They inspected the effects of adjunctive VNS more than two years in this patient populace. Grown-up outpatients with an eternal or intermittent significant burdensome issue or bipolar (I or II) issue and encountering a treatment-resistant, non-psychotic MDE (DSM-IV criteria) got two years of VNS.

Changes in psychotropic prescriptions and VNS improvement parameters were permitted simply after the initial three months.

The reaction was characterized as more noteworthy than or equivalent to a 50% decrease from the benchmark 28-item Hamilton Rating Scale for Depression (HAM-D-28) all out score, and the reduction was characterized as a HAM-D-28 score not exactly or equivalent to 10.

In light of the last perception conveyed forward investigations, HAM-D-28 reaction rates were 31% (18/59) following three months, 44% (26/59) following one year, and 42% (25/59) following two years of adjunctive VNS. Abatement rates were 15% (9/59) at 3 months, 27% (16/59) at 1 year, and 22% (13/59) at 2 years.

By two years, two passing (inconsequential to VNS) had happened, four members had pulled back from the examination, and 81% (48/59) were all the while getting VNS. Longer-term VNS was, for the most part, well-tolerated.

These examiners presumed that their discoveries propose that patients with continuous or repetitive, TRD may show long-term advantage when treated with VNS.

George et al. (2005) expressed that past reports had depicted the effects of VNS in addition to the treatment of course (VNS+TAU) during open preliminaries of patients with TRD.

To more readily comprehend these effects on the long-term result, these analysts contrasted 12month VNS+TAU results and those of a similar TRD gathering. Confirmation criteria were comparable for those getting VNS+TAU (n = 205) or just TAU (n = 124).

In the essential investigation, repeated-measures straight relapse was utilized to look at the VNS+TAU gathering (month to month information) with the TAU gathering (quarterly report) as per scores of the 30-item Inventory of Depressive Symptomatology-Self-Report (IDSSR(30)).

The two gatherings had comparative gauge statistic information, mental and treatment accounts, and degrees of treatment opposition, then again, actually more TAU members had in any event ten earlier significant burdensome scenes, and the VNS+TAU bunch had progressively electroconvulsive treatment before study section.

The VNS+TAU bunch was related with more noteworthy improvement every month in IDS-SR(30) than the TAU bunch crosswise over a year ($p < 0.001$).

Reaction rates as per the 24-item Hamilton Rating Scale for Depression (the last perception conveyed forward) at a year were 27% for the VNS+TAU gathering and 13% for the TAU gathering ($p < 0.011$). The two groups got comparative TAU (drugs and electroconvulsive treatment) during follow-up.

These examiners presumed that this correlation of 2 comparative yet non-randomized TRD bunches indicated that VNS+TAU was related with a unique anti-depressant advantage for more than a year.

These fundamental discoveries by Nahas et al. (2005), just as George as et (2005) should be approved by imminent, randomized placebo-controlled thinks about.

In a randomized controlled 10-week investigation, Rush and partners (2005a) contrasted adjunctive VNS and hoax treatment in 235 outpatients with non-psychotic significant burdensome issues ($n = 210$) or non-psychotic, discouraged stage, bipolar issue ($n = 25$). Subjects had not reacted satisfactorily to between 2 to 6 research-qualified drug preliminaries.

A 2-week, single-blind recuperation period (no stimulation) and afterwards, ten weeks of covered dynamic or hoax VNS pursued implantation.

Meds were kept stable. Essential efficacy result among 222 evaluable members depended on reaction rates (more prominent than or equivalent to 50% decrease from the pattern on the 24-item Hamilton Rating Scale for Depression [HRSD (24)]).

At 10 weeks, the response to HRSD (24) was 15.2% (n = 112) for the active group and 10% (n = 110) for the placebo group (p = 0.251).

Besides, the BlueCross BlueShield TEC appraisal on VNS for TRD (2005) expressed that this strategy doesn't meet the TEC criteria.

The TEC evaluation expressed that the accessible proof is insufficient to allow finishes of the effect of VNS treatment on wellbeing results.

As indicated by the TEC appraisal, "the accessible proof comprises of a case arrangement of 60 patients getting VNS, a short-term (i.e., 3-month) randomized, sham-controlled clinical preliminary of 221 patients, and an observational investigation contrasting 205 patients on VNS treatment compared with 124 patients accepting progressing treatment for wretchedness.

Patients who reacted to hoax treatment in the short-term randomized, controlled preliminary (roughly 10%) were barred from the long-term observational investigation. The quiet choice was a worry for all examinations.

VNS is proposed for treatment-refractory melancholy, yet the section criteria of the disappointment of 2 medications and a 6-week preliminary of treatment may not be a severe enough meaning of treatment obstruction.

Treatment refractory misery ought to be characterized by exhaustive state-of-the-art mental assessment and the board".

The BlueCross BlueShield Association refreshed their evaluation in August 2006 and presumed that VNS doesn't meet the TEC criteria.

The evaluation clarified that "[s]ince the last TEC Assessment, there have been no investigations announcing clinical results on any new or different patients. Information from the case arrangement and clinical preliminaries have been reanalyzed to show what extents of patients who react at one time are still responders at the following time point.

Nonetheless, this data independent from anyone else doesn't give proof of the efficacy of VNS past that provided by the first observational examination of VNS versus treatment not surprisingly."

An appraisal of VNS for extreme misery by the Aggressive Research Intelligence Facility (ARIF, 2005) expressed: "To finish up, this is an experimental and so far doubtful strategy for treatment for serious melancholy.

If this treatment is used, patients ought to be instructed concerning the innovative idea of the procedure and ought to be evaluated by a specialist in the field, who knows about the treatment. The treatment ought to preferably be given as a significant aspect of an authoritative assessment of clinical effectiveness and wellbeing to add to the existing proof base". Besides, an evaluation by California.

Innovation Assessment Forum (CTAF, 2006) reasoned that the utilization of VNS for the treatment of safe discouragement doesn't meet CTAF's innovation evaluation criteria for wellbeing, effectiveness, and improvement in wellbeing results.

A specialist expressed that VNS is another methodology in treating neuropsychiatric infections inside the class of brain-stimulating gadgets known as neuromodulators.

Even though VNS has gotten FDA endorsement for the treatment of medication-resistant discouragement,there is an absence of Class I proof of effectiveness in treating melancholy. The creators presumed considerably more research is required concerning precisely how to refine and convey the electrical heartbeats and how this differentially affects mind work in wellbeing and illness.

The Centers for Medicare also Medicaid Services (CMS, 2007) expressed that there is sufficient proof to presume that VNS isn't sensible and essential for the treatment of safe discouragement. Accordingly, CMS has declared a national non-coverage assurance for this sign.

In a regular audit on the wellbeing and effectiveness of VNS in the administration of patients with TRD, Daban and associates (2008) presumed that VNS is by all accounts a fascinating new way to deal with treating TRD.

Be that as it may, notwithstanding the promising outcomes detailed chiefly in open investigations, further clinical preliminaries are essential to affirm its effectiveness insignificant sadness.

Also, contemplates on its instrument of activity and cost-effectiveness are additionally expected to comprehend and create VNS treatment for affective issue all the more likely.

This is in concurrence with the perception of Fitzgerald and Daskalakis (2008), who expressed that given the intrusive idea of VNS and potential side effects, further research on its utilization for the treatment of sorrow is earnestly required.

This ought to incorporate the advancement of indicators of clinical reaction and meaning of stimulation parameters with upgraded effectiveness.

An Agency for Healthcare Research and Quality's audit detailed that there is insufficient proof to assess whether non-pharmacological medications are effective for TRD. The audit condensed proof of the effectiveness of 4 non-pharmacological medicines:

i. electroconvulsive treatment (ECT),
ii. dreary transcranial attractive stimulation (rTMS),
iii. VNS, and
iv. subjective social treatment (CBT) or relational psychotherapy.

As for looking after abatement (or anticipating backslide), there were no immediate examinations (proof), including ECT, rTMS, VNS, or CBT.

As to a total proof, there were three reasonable preliminaries contrasted, rTMS and a trick methodology, and they found no noteworthy differences. In any case, not many patients were pursued during the backslide counteractive action stages in 2 of the three investigations (20week and 6-month follow-up), and patients in the third examination (3month follow-up) got a co-intervention giving insufficient proof to an end.

There were no qualified investigations for ECT, VNS, or, on the other hand, psychotherapy.

The survey inferred that that similar clinical research on non-pharmacologic mediations in a TRD populace is right off the bat in its prime stages, and numerous clinical inquiries regarding efficacy and effectiveness stay unanswered. Understanding of the information is considerably ruined by differing meanings of TRD and the lack of pertinent examinations.

The best volume of proof is for ECT and rTMS. In any case, in any event, for a couple of examinations of medicines that are bolstered by some evidence, the quality of proof is low for benefits, reflecting little certainty that the proof mirrors the genuine effect and showing that further research is probably going to change our trust in these discoveries.

This finding of low quality is generally prominent in 2 cases: ECT and rTMS didn't deliver different clinical results in TRD, and ECT created preferred effects over pharmacotherapy. No preliminaries legitimately looked at the probability of keeping up reduction for non-pharmacologic mediations.

A couple of preliminaries tending to unfavourable occasions, subpopulations, subtypes, and health-related results gave low or insufficient proof of differences between non-pharmacologic mediations.

The direst subsequent stages for inquiring about are to apply a predictable meaning of TRD, to direct more head-to-head clinical preliminaries contrasting non-pharmacologic intercessions and themselves and with pharmacologic medications, and to outline the quantity of treatment disappointments following a treatment endeavor of sufficient portion and span in the present scene cautiously.

As of late, VNS has been utilized to treat patients with a chemical imbalance, weight, Alzheimer's sickness, and obsessive-compulsive issue. Results from pilot ponders recommended that VNS may prompt weight reduction in vast people and improve individual capacity in patients with Alzheimer's ailment. In any case, these discoveries should be approved in huge randomized placebo-controlled thinks about long-term results.

In an open-label study, Camilleri and partners evaluated the effects of vagal blocking by methods for another therapeutic gadget that utilizations high-frequency electrical calculations to make irregular vagal blocking (VBLOC treatment) on overabundance weight reduction (EWL).

Anodes were embedded laparoscopically on the two vagi close to the esophagogastric intersection to give an electrical square. Patients (stout subjects with weight list [BMI] of 35 to 50 kg/m(2)) were pursued for a half year for body weight, security, electrocardiogram, dietary admission, satiation, satiety, and pancreatic plasma polypeptide (PP) reaction to hoax sustaining.

To explicitly evaluate gadget effects alone, no eating routine or exercise programs were established. A sum of 31 patients (mean BMI, 41.2 +/- 1.4 kg/m(2)) got the gadget. Mean EWL at 4 as well as 12 weeks and a half year after embed was 7.5%, 11.6%, and 14.2%, separately (all $p < 0.001$); 25% of patients lost more than 25% EWL at a half year (most extreme, 36.8%).

There were no passings or device-related certain antagonistic occasions (AEs). Calorie consumption diminished by more prominent than 30% at 4 and 12 weeks and a half year (all $p <$ or $= 0.01$), with prior satiation ($p < 0.001$) and decreased appetite ($p = 0.005$). Following 12 weeks, plasma PP reactions were smothered (20 +/- 7 versus 42 +/- 19 pg/ml).

Normal percent EWL in patients with PP reaction under 25 pg/ml was twofold that with PP reaction more prominent than 25 pg/ml ($p = 0.02$).

Three patients had genuine AEs that necessary brief hospitalization, one each for the lower respiratory tract, subcutaneous embed site seroma, and clostridium difficile the runs.

The creators presumed that VBLOC treatment is related with huge EWL and an alluring wellbeing profile. They noticed that these discoveries have brought about the structure and execution of a randomized, double-blind, planned, multi-centre preliminary in a broad subject populace.

Vagal nerve stimulation is additionally being read for treating constant cerebral pains; be that as it may, its incentive for this sign still can't seem to be built up.

It was accounted for that VNS was embedded in 4 men and two ladies with the debilitating interminable group and headache migraines.

Two persistent migraine patients showed major headaches change. In 5 patients, the treatment was well-tolerated, whereas 1 had nausea, including at the lowest relative strength.

VGN for Better Digestion

Have you ever heard of the nerve of the vagus? If you have digestive problems, you should get to know it very well. A big nerve acts as a bridge from the brain to the stomach, so if you've previously heard of the mind-gut link, this is it.

In reality, digestion starts in the brain through the vagus nerve, way before food actually enters the mouth and the breakdown process begins.

It is the role of the vagus nerve which starts in the brain to facilitate the contraction of smooth contractions around the GI tract, allowing the release of gastric juices to reach the body in preparation for food.

Part of the parasympathetic nervous system, or our "rest and digest condition," is designed to help us get the digestive process going and done properly.

Yet stress, triggering cravings and more intense symptoms of hunger, can also activate the vagus nerve. So if you're like me a stress eater, that's exactly what's going on, but that's not usual.

The explanation of why this is so critical is that if the brain misfires messages to the vagus nerve, such as when under chronic stress, the whole gastrointestinal system can be disrupted. We stop producing sufficient bile levels (which are needed to break down fats), the smooth muscles around our GI tract are not beginning to contract on time, and we are not entering the rest and digest process properly.

This can induce hypermotility, or "gastric dumping" (rapid bowel emptying), resulting in malabsorption and malnutrition, including more serious issues such as autoimmune conditions and IBD.

Therefore, you need to take care of your vagus nerve to better fix cravings, changes in appetite, and ensure that you are completely in a state of rest and digestion when you feed!

Now you probably think: "How much do I know about a particular nerve in my body?!"In addition, there are some very easy things that you can do that will help you far beyond digestion.

Because this nerve transports so much blood all over the body, it also plays an important role in immune function. So you should defer to those of you with an autoimmune disease like me!

These tips will also help you respond better and cope with stress, which will take off your adrenal glands a huge load!

Oxytocin, or our brain's "feel good" chemical, can help regulate normal vagus nerve activity and keep digestion under control. Here are a couple of ways to boost or stimulate the production of oxytocin: eat right now.

Take a few long breaths, put your phone away, and get present before you take a little food. This will have direct benefits in terms of sleep and stress relief.

There's acupuncture. Let's get back the nice flow of energy!

Via reflection. This alone will activate the parasympathetic nervous system, and it only takes 5-20 minutes a day to do so!

Laughter, Laughter. How quick is it?! To call a good friend, to watch a comedy show or to play with a child is likely to result in laughter.

Exercise. It raises the levels of oxytocin and serotonin.

Therapies for mental and calming. If you want to dig deeper, there are many choices here. Ask your local health center or hospital for massage.

Good healthy fats: fish oil, olive oil, EPA and DHA all encourage vagus nerve stimulation you will also want to make careful that no external factors interfere with the development of oxytocin and activation of the vagus nerve.

A few things to remember: are you actually exposed to any materials, dirt, molds, liquids, gases, or radiation?

Have you been previously exposed to any toxins?

Have you ever needed to take food from a source you aren't too sure of how healthy it is?

Do you currently have anything unusual in your life that can affect your health status positively or negatively?

Have you undergone any big changes in your life? (e.g., traveling, changing jobs, changing marriages, death, etc.)

However, if you've been struggling with digestive problems for a while, it may be time to assess whether any of the aforementioned causes are absent and think about how you can infuse them more into your life.

ROLE OF VAGAL & SPINAL SENSORY PATHWAYS ON ECC'S ACTIVITY

In the regulation of eupneic diaphragmatic activity, the relationships between vagal and spinal afferents are observed in two classes of cats anesthetized with either pentobarbital sodium (SPB) or even with ethyl carbamate-alpha-chloralose (ECC), that improved spinal reflexes.

Two research procedures are conducted within both types of anesthesia:

1. bilateral cervical vagotomy accompanied by C8-level spinal section or
2. spinal section accompanied by vagotomy.

During eupneic ventilation as well as tracheal occlusion at the end of the expiration, improvements in integrated diaphragmatic behavior (Edi) are observed.

Vagotomy has always significantly increased the magnitude of Edi during eupnea (SPB + 30%; ECC + 15%) as well as expanded its length (Tdi) (SPB + 110%; ECC + 75%) but has not altered the overall shape of the Edi vs. time relationship.

The spinal segment caused reverse shifts in Edi's amplitude, if vagal afferents are present or blocked, and altered the Edi wave's structure, which did not alter Tdi substantially.

Such results show that both vagal, as well as spinal afferents, might be involved in regulating eupneic motivation but have distinct and interrelated effects on phrenic motoneuron selection and firing time.

In fact, under ECC anesthesia, Tdi measured throughout tracheal occlusion (Todi) became greatly increased.

Todi that became similar to the standards acquired in intact or spinal cats during SPB anesthesia decreased in this circumstance spinal segment.

Hence the end-expiration reaction to tracheal occlusion can never be understood as a consequence of the mere repression of volume-related vagal data.

VAGUS NERVE AS MODULATOR OF BRAIN-GUT AXIS

The vagus nerve is the main part of the parasympathetic system, which controls a wide range of vital body functions such as mood control, immune response, metabolism, as well as heart rate.

It defines one of the links between both the brain and the gastrointestinal tract and directs sensory information via afferent fibers about the state of the internal organs.

In this review part, we would discuss more about the vagus nerve's various functions that make it an attractive destination for psychiatric as well as gastrointestinal disorders treatment.

There is decent evidence that activation of the vagus nerve is a promising potential therapy for medication-refractory anxiety, post-traumatic stress disorder as well as inflammatory disease of the intestine.

Treatments aimed at the vagus nerve hike vagal tone and also inhibit the production of cytokine. Both of these are essential resilience mechanisms.

Stimulating vagal afferent fibers in the intestine affects monoaminergic brain networks in the brainstem that play critical roles in various psychiatric conditions, including mood and also anxiety.

In particular, there is research indicating that intestinal bacteria have beneficial effects on mood as well as anxiety, partially by influencing the vagus nerve function.

Since the vagal tone is associated with the ability to control stress responses and it can be affected by breathing, its development by meditation and yoga is likely to contribute to tolerance and reduction of symptoms of mood and anxiety.

Introduction

In order to regulate gastrointestinal homeostasis and relate psychological to cognosis, the bi-directional interaction between a brain and a gastrointestinal tract, recognized as the brain-gooled axis, is based upon the complex system of the vagus nerve, but it is also sympathetic (e.g., prevertebral ganglia), endocrine, immune, humoral connections and the impact of gut microbiota.

The ENS contains about 30 neurotransmitters and has more receptors than the backbone.

Blood-brain boundary (e.g., ghrelin) crosses chemicals and peptides that the ENS releases into the blood circulation and synergistically works with the vagus nerve, for instance, to regulate food intake and appetite.

As a treatment target of digestive and psychiatric disorders, including inflammatory bowel disease, anxiety, and post-traumatic stress (PTSD), the brain-good axis is becoming increasingly important.

The intestine is an important control center of the immune system and has immunomodulative characteristics.

This nerve, therefore, plays a major role in the connection between the intestines, the heart, and inflammation.

Of starters, vagus nerve stimulation (VNS) and meditation techniques are new treatment methods of modulating the brain-good axis.

These treatments proved beneficial to mood and anxiety disorders but also to increased inflammation under other conditions.

In particular, gut-directed bowel syndrome and IBD hypnotherapy are shown to be successful.

The vagus nerve is also an important link between diet and psychological, neurological, and inflammatory diseases.

The Vagus Nerve manipulates your hunger level

Hunger and fullness signals are a really essential form of interaction that flows up and down the vagus nerve. The bodily bulk of meals in the stomach, for example, sends hunger or satiety signals to your brain from the vagus nerve. This is how the brain knows that after a meal you can stop feeling thirsty.

Sensing of nutrients, including neurotransmitters released in the intestine, such as serotonin as well as ghrelin, may also send signals of appetite and fullness to the brain.

Obesity is correlated with lower responsiveness of the vagus nerve to signals of fullness, and there is a great deal of proof to show that it is caused by diet in particular.

Obesity-inducing diets will actually change the response of just the vagus nerve to fullness stimuli, and making the "full now" message takes more fuel for your brain.

But as you might expect, activating the vagus nerve (to "turn the volume" on the satiety signal) in laboratory animals usually causes weight loss–although it is important to note that observational studies have mixed results.

Hunger's Vagus Nerve and many other health problems are important reasons why the vagus nerve is essential. But if you skyrocket to PubMed, you will discover that vagus nerve disorder is necessarily associated with other problems of all kinds.

This is because the vagus nerve as well helps regulate inflammation, as well as every chronic disease involves inflammation.

Anti-inflammatory is the activation of vagus nerve impulses to the brain–this allows the brain to reject the stress response as well as reduce the development of inflammatory cytokines.

The results here are a bit difficult to untangle even though the vagus nerve is a two-way street because there are a lot of complex feedback loops between both the brain and the intestine (actually recall the vagus nerve goes both ways!).

But the exact mechanism may be less important for people who care about enhancing their wellbeing than the outcomes, which are undoubtedly impressive: vagus nerve regulation of inflammation influences cardiovascular health, as well as vagus nerve stimulation, can help to prevent cardiovascular issues.

In patients with Crohn's Disease (a type of Inflammatory Bowel Disease) vagus nerve signalling is thrown off, and a small preliminary study showed that vagal nerve stimulation tends to treat the cause.

For Irritable Bowel Syndrome, the vagus nerve could also be involved, and vagal stimulation may be helpful in reducing IBS discomfort.

This experiment is really interesting: both anxiety and insulin resistance was avoided by curing rats prone to diabetes with vagal nerve stimulation.

This is a germaine line of proof that both anxiety and diabetes may have origins in the stomach.

If a bad diet affects the vagus nerve's resistance, it may also affect both of these diseases in the second hand.

This might be one justification why in overall health, gut health is just such a major player.

So far, we learn that an obesogenic "cafeteria diet" (high-fat, high-carb junk food) lowers the vagus nerve's resistance, and also that vagus nerve stimulation mitigates this, with great benefits for weight... and for almost everything else.

Sadly, in these experiments, "vagal nerve stimulation" is not something that you can do at home; it is a tool that has been implanted in these bodies by the participants.

But if the vagus nerve's sensitivity can be reduced by a lousy diet, perhaps a good diet helps restore it. Apart from "don't eat a diet of junk food," here is a bit more precise work.

This study found inflammation decreased by dietary fat through its impact on the nerve of the vagus.

The researchers noted that "high-fat... nutrition is conceivably therapeutic in various inflammatory diseases such as sepsis as well as inflammatory bowel disease (IBD) typified by an inflammatory response in which... intestinal barrier function is impaired."

This is supported by the association between a ketogenic (very high-fat, low-carb) diet as well as vagal nerve stimulation as two effective therapies.

A ketogenic diet will have some of the anti-inflammatory, hunger-suppressing benefits by activating your vagus nerve.

This study also showed that the vagus nerve was activated by a probiotic (which is Lactobacillus casei strain Shirota).

For students taking a challenging test, the probiotic changed the gut-to-brain pressure signalling and reduced the output of the stress hormone cortisol.

It indicates that probiotics may break the cycle of gut-brain-gut-brain input around and around the vagus nerve, where psychological distress causes trouble in the heart, which sends more signs of hormonal stress to the brain, causing more trouble in the gut.

Aerobics can be helpful as well.

You could also use the Valsalva maneuver to conduct all your vagal nerve stimulation for immediate gratification. Sit down, it can render you really dizzy. Breathe deeply, then shut the lips and pinch the nose such that no air may escape.

Then say you're gasping for air out, but you must feel pressure from the breeze without raising the nose or mouth.

Try to do it for 15-20 seconds, and let the air outside and breathe normally. (If you do a little weightlifting, this is the kind of breath-holding that you do to balance your back during hard squats and deadlifts.) The Valsalva maneuver does not have long-term effects but may be useful for a situation at hand, just before an exam or in the midst of a tense flow.

That's not much to go on with –there's just not a lot of food and vagus nerve trials. Yet beginning with it is essential, and it confirms the significant ways that the heart, the brain, as well as the other parts of your body are all linked.

Understanding the vagus nerve goes some way to explaining why gut health, mental health, and the health of the whole body are so tangled together, as well as why good gut health is so essential for things that go beyond digestion.

ANATOMY OF THE VAGUS NERVE

The vagus nerve transmits the brain and vice versa with a wide variety of stimuli from the digestive system as well as lungs.

It is the 10th cranium nerve that passes from its origin in the brainstem through the chest and thorax to the abdomen. Because of its long journey through the human body, it was also known as the "wanderer nerve."

In the groove corresponding to the olive and the lower peduncle of the brain, the vagus nerve enters the medulla oblongata and exits the skull in the centre of the jugular foramen.

For most pharynx and larynx muscles, which are responsible for swallowing and vocalizing, the vagus nerve in the neck provides ample innervation.

This provides the heart in the thorax with the largest parasympathetic source and induces a decrease in heart rate. In the intestines, the vagus nerve regulates the smooth movement of the muscle and glandular development.

Vagal efferent neurons arise from the vagus nerve's dorsal motor nucleus in the medulla and interview the muscle and mucosal surfaces of the intestine in both the lamina propria and external muscularis.

The celiac section feeds the intestine from the proximal duodenum to the distal part of the descending colon.

The abdominal vagal afferents include mucosal mechanoreceptors, pharmacopoieceticals, and voltage receptors in an esophagus, stomachs and proximal small intestines, and sensory endings in the liver and pancreas.

The sensory afferent cell bodies in the Nodose Ganglia relay inputs to the Nukleus tractos solitarii (NTS) systems to several vagal sensory data CNS areas, such as the locus coeruleus (LC), rostral ventrolateral medulla, amygdala, as well as thalamus.

Definition of the anatomy of the vagus nerve.

The vagus nerve controls internal brain processes such as appetite, heart rate, and breath rate, as well as movement of the vasomotor and certain involuntary acts such as vomiting, sneezing, and swallowing.

The activation allows for the development of acetylcholine (ACh) at the synaptic junction of secrant cells, nerve fibers, and smooth muscles. ACh binds in the parasympathetic nervous system with nicotinic and muscarinic receptors and induces muscle contractions.

Animal studies have shown an impressive regeneration of the vagus nerve. For instance, subdiaphragmatic vagotomy lead to the movement and regeneration of central vagal afferents, as well as synaptic plasticity in the NTS.

In contrast, vagal afferent reconstruction can be performed in rats 18 weeks after subdiaphragmatic vagotomy, even though the gastrointestinal tract regeneration outbreak is not resolved until 45 weeks after additional Vagus nerve stimulation operates by adding electrical impulses to the vagus nerve.

This functions to activate the vagus nerve. The activation of the vagus nerve can be done in two different ways: a direct invasive stimulation that is actually the most common procedure and an indirect non-invasive transcutaneous stimulation.

Invasive VNS (iVNS) requires subcutaneous implantation of a small pulse generator into the left thoracic region. Electrodes are attached to the nerve of the left cervical vagus and connected to the pulse generator by a plume under the body.

The motor transmits through the vagus nerve transient electrical impulses to the heart. These electrical impulses are thought to have antiepileptic, therapeutic, and anti-inflammatory effects by altering the excitability of the nerve cell.

Transcutaneous VNS (TVNS) promotes non-invasive stimulation of the vagus nerve without surgery, in contrast to iVNS.

In this case, throughout the subcutaneous course of just the afferent auricular nervous branch, the stimulator is usually connected to the auricular concha through ear clips and provides electrical momentum.

For 30–37 percent of patients, a pilot study investigating the use of VNS for 60 patients with therapy-resistant depressive disorders showed significant medical progress and high tolerability.

Five years later, the US was able to relieve refractory anxiety by relaxing the vagus nerve. Food and Drug Administration (FDA).

Since then, as can be seen below, many observational studies have shown the safety and efficacy of VNS in anxiety. For contrast, no controlled placebo-control clinical study consistently shows beneficial effects of VNS.

The neural role of VNS is unclear and therefore needs further research to understand whether VNS will help patients who do not respond to conventional antidepressants.

Neuroimaging behavioral studies have shown that VNS affects the roles of several cortical and subcortical regions. Through direct or indirect neural connections via NTS, the vagus nerve has biological interactions with a number of moods, affecting limbic and prefrontal brain areas.

Therefore, PET experiments studies show resting brain function in the ventromedial prefrontal cortex (vmPFC) reduces, which is intended to modulate stress in chronic VNS for anxiety by the amygdala and other brain regions.

In these regions, VNS leads to chemical changes in the synthesis of monoamines and antidepressant activity.

The association regarding monoamine and antidepressant activity has been shown by different types of research. In the synaptic break, both monoamine-increasing drugs — serotonin (5-HT), NE, or dopamine (DA)—have antidepressant effects.

Therefore, the loss of monoamines contributes to depressive symptoms in people with an elevated risk of depression.

Chronic VNS influences brain and blood fluid levels of 5-HT, NE, and DA. In rats, it is proven that VNS therapies cause significant changes in basal neuronal activity in serotonin's brainstem nuclei in the dorsal raphe nucleus encourage long-term dependency.

Therefore, chronic VNS was associated with increased levels of dorsal raphe serotonin extracellular.

Different evidence suggests that NE in the pathophysiology and diagnosis of depressive disorders is a significant neurotransmitter.

In fact, an unexplained weakening of NE in the brain led to a return to depressive symptoms after a completed treatment with NE antidepressant drugs.

The LC comprises the highest population of noradrenergic neurons in the brain as well as receives NTS projections that are backed up by the vagus nerve in turn.

VNS thereby enhances the NE neuronal firing rate and thus increases the serotonin neuronal firing frequency.

Therefore, it was shown that the amount of NE in the prefrontal cortex increased. The noradrenergy neuron pharmacological damage caused the loss of VNS effects.

With respect to DA, it has been shown that the short-term (14 days) and long-term (12 months) effects of VNS in major immune depression can contribute to a brainstem dopaminergic stimulus.

DA is a catecholamine that is synthesized exclusively in the intestine and plays a crucial role in the reward process of the brain.

In fact, it is possible to exert monoamine-independently positive effects of VNS. VNS treatment may, therefore, lead to dynamic shifts in hippocampal monoamine metabolites, and many studies have documented the impact of VNS on neurogenesis in the hippocampus.

This cycle was considered an essential mechanism of physiology for maintaining normal moods.

Serotonin is also an active neurotransmitter in the intestine, which activates the vagus nerve and causes nausea and vomiting to cause peristalsis.

Therefore, it is necessary to control vital functions such as appetite but also sleep, contributing to feelings of well-being.

A type of neuroendocrine that lurks the lumen of the digestive tract next to the epithelium is formed to 95 percent of enterochromaffin cells.

In response to the mechanical or chemical stimulation of the gastrointestinal tract, serotonin is released from enterochromaffin cells leading to the activation of 5-HT3 receptors in the vagal afferent terminals. There are also 5-HT3 receptors, like afferent neurons in the gastrointestinal vagus, in the soma in which 5-HT can be activated.

There are also 5-HT3 receptors in the central terminals of vagal afferents that function to enhance glutamatergic synaptic transmission to second-order nucleus tractus solitarius neurons within the brainstem.

As a result, associations in the stomach and brain between the vagus nerve and serotonin processes tend to play an important role in psychiatric treatment.

Vagus-Related Treatment of Depression

Pathophysiology of acute anxiety. Major depressive malfunction is one of the leading causes of worldwide disease burden. With a lifetime rate of 1.0 percent (Czech Republic) to 16.9 percent (US), the cost of poverty poses a significant economic burden on our society.

Depression pathophysiology is nuanced and includes external contextual stresses; genetic and biochemical mechanisms such as monamine neurotransmission overdrive of the HPA axis, inflammation, and diseases as mentioned above.

For example, a shortage of serotonin-precursor tryptophan amino acid can trigger depressive symptoms such as mood loss, anxiety, and desperation.

Overdriven HPA axis is most often seen in people with severe (i.e., melancholic or psychotic) anxiety when cortisol feedback inhibitory pathways become compromised due to cytokine over-secretion.

It is proven that prolonged exposure to high inflammatory cytokines leads to depression (108). This may be expatiated by the fact that cytokine overexpression results in a fall in serotonin levels.

Therefore, anti-inflammatory treatment has the ability to reduce the symptoms of depression. Specifically, IBD is an important risk factor for mood and anxiety disorders, increasing the risk of IBD exacerbation.

The European multicenter study found a positive effect of VNS on depressive symptoms in people with therapy-resistant depression.

The 3-month VNS rollout resulted in a response rate of 37% and a remission rate of 17%. After a year of treatment, the rate of response was 53%, and the remission rate was 33%.

A meta-analysis comparing the use of VNS with usual treatment for depressed patients observed an acute response rate of about 50 percent and a 20 percent long-term remission rate after 2 years of treatment. Several other studies have also shown increased long-term benefits of VNS for depression-resistant clinical therapy.

By comparison, a 5-year longitudinal observational study comparing drug effects as normal and VNS as an additional approach to usual treatment only for therapy-resistant depression found a higher medical benefit and a higher level of rehabilitation in the VNS family.

This also applies to patients with co-morbid depression and anxiety that often fail to respond to studies of antidepressants. These were all open-label studies and did not use a randomized, placebo-controlled study design.

It is important to note that people with anxiety have high concentrations of cerebrospinal fluid in serum and proinflammatory cytokines.

The benefit of VNS in depression could be due to the inhibitory effect of the synthesis of proinflammatory cytokines and a marked increase of peripheral anti-inflammatory circulatory cytokines.

On the other hand, improvement after VNS has been associated with modified CRH secretion to prevent overdriving the HPA axis. A direct stimulating effect transfer from the vagus nerve through the NTS to the paraventricular nucleus of the hypothalamus may result in altered development and secretion of CRH.

Eventually, the development of TNF-α peripheral blood, which is elevated in clinical depression, has been shown to be suppressed.

Immune and nervous systems may be impaired by intestinal microbiota in the role of diet depressive effects. This may lead to a greater improvement in the mental effects of people who are anxious or nervous.

There is increasing evidence that by interacting with intestinal microbiota, nutritional components such as probiotics, gluten, and drugs such as antioxidants and antibiotics have a strong impact on the activity of the vagus nerve.

In addition, animal studies have shown that the vagus nerve is involved in microbiota contact with the brain and that interaction can contribute to relaxation and actions.

For example, Lactobacillus species have gained considerable attention due to their use of probiotics and the promotion of their health.

Bravo et al. showed that chronic treatment of mice with Lactobacillus rhamnosus (strainJB-1) caused lower levels of stress-induced corticosterones and similar behavior to anxiety and depression.

Chronic L diagnosis has been shown. Induced regional-dependent GABA(B1b) mRNA changes in the brain with increases in cortical (cenulate and pre-limbic) regions and concomitant decreases in signals of hippocampus, amygdala and LC.

Therefore, in the prefrontal cortex and amygdala, L. GABA(Aα2) mRNA expression has been reduced by rhamnosus(JB-1), but by GABA(Aα2) boosted in the hippocampus, reversing a common phenotype of depressive symptoms: loss of prefrontal regulation and overaction in subcortic and anxiogenic brain regions.

Significantly, L. Rhamnosis (JB-1) reduced corticosterone-induced stress and anxiety-and depression-related behavior. This cannot be alarming because changes in the core expression of GABA receptors are implicated in the pathogenesis of anxiety and depression.

L's anxiety and calming effect. Rhamnosus was not found in vagotomized mice to identify the vagus as a major modulatory constitutive medium for communication in the gut and brain between the exposed bacteria.

Accordingly, the anxiolytic effect of Bifidobacterium longum therapy in mice that were vagotomized before colitis was caused was absent in a model of anxiety-like colitis.

In humans, owing to their antidepressant and anxiolytic activity, a class of anti-inflammatory probiotics may be effective in treating patients with psychiatric disorders.

Differences in intestinal microbiota makeup have been shown in people who experience relative anxiety with healthy people.

Importantly, this resulted in suicidal actions to collect fecal samples from five depressed patients into germ-free mice.

Effect of depression relaxation techniques. It has been shown that love-childhood counseling self-generated positive emotions lead to an increase in positive emotions compared to the control group, an effect moderated by the clear vagal tone.

In addition, elevated positive emotions have produced improvements in vagal tone that are likely affected by improved social interaction expectations.

Insomnia, depression, and chronic pain people have been routinely practiced for rehabilitation, showing a significant improvement in symptom severity.

Controlled studies have found methods focused on yoga to be effective in treating symptoms of depression from mildly depressed to severe depressive (MDD).

Some yoga exercises specifically activate the vagus nerve by elevating the vagal tone, which enhances independent control, cognitive functions, and mood and stress regulation.

The suggested neurophysiological pathways for yoga-based therapy effectiveness in alleviating depression symptoms indicate that yoga breathing leads to higher vagal tones.

Many studies explain the influence of yogic breathing on brain function and physiological parameters.

Sudarshan Kriya Yoga (SKY), a form of relaxation therapy, stimulates the fuzzy nerve and has numerous independent impacts, including changes in heart rate and increased memory and bowel function.

The series of different breathing techniques of end-inspiration and end-expiratory grips create different signals during SKY from several tactile afferents, sensory receptors, and baroreceptors.

These are likely to affect different vaginal tissues, resulting in physiological changes in the lungs and influencing the limbic system.

Recent research deducted that even patients who did not respond to antidepressants showed a significant reduction in signs of depression and anxiety compared to the control group following 8 weeks of direct SKY treatment.

Iyengar yoga showed reduced depression symptoms in subjects.

Iyengar yoga is related to increased HRV, supporting the theory that yoga breathing and postures partly work with an increased tone of parasympathy.

Vagus-Related Treatment of PSD

Post-traumatic stress disorder is a condition of depression following injuries that is characterized by intrusive visions, delusions, hyper-vigilance, agitation, emotional alienation, and social disorder.

Using the DSM-5 definition, it has an 8.3% lifetime rate. Signs of PTSD can be classified into four clusters: signs of pain, avoidance, psychological and affective changes, and anticipatory and responsive rises.

Those with PTSD tend to live as if they were compromised chronically. They show battle and flight behaviour or chronic personality collapse and dissociation, no likelihood of a calm state and positive social interaction.

With time, these independent maladaptive responses can result in an increased risk of psychiatric comorbidity such as dependence or cardiovascular disease.

Post-traumatic stress disorder symptoms are partly mediated by the vagus nerve. There is data of PTSD of diminished parasympathetic activity that indicates an individual discrepancy.

Vagal heart rate control varies with ingestion by myelinated vagal fibers.

Therefore, by quantifying the amplitude of rhythmic heart rate fluctuations–respiratory sinus arrhythmia (RSA), the vagal influence on the heart can be calculated.

A recent study of PTSD vets showed a decrease in RSA rest. By contrast, with healthy controls, patients with PTSD reported greater variation by heart rate in high-frequency relative.

One of many PTSD features is the continuous display of conditioned stimuli's physiological responses despite the absence of acute injury.

Behavioral therapies used to control PTSD rely on helping the patient to gradually reduce their fear of this symbol over time.

Therefore, the gold standard for PTSD therapy is considered to be exposure-based therapies.

The goal of exposure-based treatment is to substitute associations with chronic stress with new, more acceptable associations relative to nervous associations.

Research has deduced that individuals with PTSD have the network of fear extinction with low elimination and defective activation.

This network includes the vmPFC, amygdala, and hippocampus. It is extremely important for the cognitive restoration of depression following extinction events.

The incidence of post-traumatic stress disorder and structural abnormalities is associated with the former hippocampus and centromedial tonsillitis. There is evidence of increased activation of amygdala during controlled fear in humans and rodents.

There are synaptic mutual relations between the amygdala and vmPFC. In fact, under conditions of uncertainty and threat, the PFC may become hypocritical, leading to the failure to inhibit amygdala overactivity, such as hyperarousal and re-experience, with the development of PTSD symptoms.

In contrast, PTSD physicians show higher basal amygdala activity during implicit facial processing in response to stressful signals as hostile gestures compared to healthy controls, as well as patients with panic disorder and generalized anxiety disorder.

As well as being an essential chunk of the anxiety loop, the hippocampus is implicated in PTSD pathophysiology.

Patients of PTSD have a smaller hippocampus density that is associated of severe symptoms. The hippocampus is a primary organ for encoding and processing episodic memory.

Hippocampal disruption contributes to human and rodent decoding deficiencies in the background. The neural network of the hippocampus, amygdala, and vmPFC is extremely important for the contextual reconstruction of post-extinction memories of fear.

Impaired hippocampal activity may lead patients to re-experience trauma symptoms, resulting in generalization of the traumatic background in patients with PTSD.

VNS in PTSD Nervous stimulation Vagus shows promise as a clinical intervention to treatment-resistant psychiatric disorders, including PTSD.

Chronic VNS has been shown to decrease anxiety in rats and increase scores in the Hamilton Anxiety Scale in people with treatment-resistant depression.

When activated, the vagus nerve sends signals to the NTS, and the NTS sends the amygdala and hypothalamus specific representations.

In comparison, VNS stimulates the development of NE in both the basolateral amygdala and hippocampus and cortex. The injection of NE amygdala contributes to a better understanding of extinction.

Therefore, VNS could be a good tool for increasing the preservation of biodiversity. Extinction, in conjunction with VNS, for example, may lead to the apprehension of regeneration and reduction of PTSD symptoms in rats.

In tandem with extinction learning, VNS stimulates the plasticity of the prefrontal infralimbian cortex and the basolateral complex of the amygdala to facilitate the reduction of conditioned threat reactions.

VNS may also improve longevity by inhibiting the activity of the sympathetic nervous system.

An abrupt decrease in VNS-induced fear would result in mortality by interfering with the sympathetic response to CS and breaking CS's relation to terror.

Nonetheless, randomized controlled trials are required for these results to be accepted.

One of the most important neurophysiological effects of VNS is to reduce hippocampal activation, probably by improving GABAergic signaling.

As a central feature of episodic memory and spatial meaning decoding, the hippocampus is a key component of the cycle of terror.

Decreased activation of the hippocampus after VNS was documented in several other studies under other conditions such as depression or schizophrenia.

Positive Nutrient Effect in PTSD Research suggests that because of stress, probiotics may have the potential to reduce inflammatory responses and associated symptoms.

An exploratory study analyzing PTSD clinicians' microbiota and untreated controls showed that three strains decreased in PTSD patients: Actinobacteria, Lentisphaerae, and Verrucomicrobia associated with higher PTSD symptoms.

A decreased overload could have caused the immune system to collapse and signs of PTSD to develop.

Studies using a murine PTSD model found that the immunization of the immunoregulatory bacterium Mycobacterium vaccae (NCTC 11659) by a heat-milled method induced a constructive behavioral response to psychosocial stress.

Healthy volunteer work has shown that specific probiotics are associated with increased well-being, decreased anxiety, and psychological distress. All of these are preliminary findings.

Well-designed, double-blind, placebo-controlled clinical studies are desperately needed to determine the effect of microbial supplementation and controlled dietary changes on the psychological symptoms and cognitive functions of patients with PTSD.

Positive Meditation and Yoga Impact on PTSD Clinical evidence was provided on the efficacy of MBSR in PTSD treatment. Sluggish breathing and long exhalation times lead to increased parasympathy for MBSR.

In fact, clinical trials showed the efficacy of yoga as a therapeutic intervention for depression and dissociation by downregulating stress response.

Following natural disasters, yoga also reduced the symptoms of PSTD. Anxiety disorders that lead to yoga, like PTSD, pair higher HRV with low GABA.

Together with the autonomous nervous system and GABA system inputs, the PFC, hippocampus, and amygdala links create a network through which yoga-based exercises can reduce symptoms.

There are indicators of PTSD that decreased amygdala activity vmPFC control is associated with impaired repression of disrupted anxiety.

Enhanced PFC activation correlated with parasympathetic behavior during yoga may improve PFC GABA projection suppression of the amygdala, decrease the overactivity of the amygdala, and minimize symptoms of PTSD.

IBD Inflammatory intestinal disease two disorders are primarily concerned with inflammatory intestinal infection: ulcerative colitis (UC) and Crohn's disease (CD).

IBD is characterized by chronic, uncontrolled gastrointestinal mucosal inflammation. Symptoms cause pain in the stomach, vomiting, fatigue, weight loss, and loss/deficiency of some body parts (skin, hair, joints).

The major signs of CD are diarrhea, abdominal pain, and weight loss, while rectal bleeding is often followed by UC diarrhea.

Inflammatory bowel diseases affect about 1.5 million people in the US and 2.2 million people in Europe, with about 20% of patients with IBD having a positive family history.

Industrialization has led to significant improvements in the level of IBD prevalence in Asia.

Environmental risk factors, including viruses, western dietary and food pollutants, air and water pollution, medications (antibiotics, hormones) and genetic stress (more than 250 genetic variables have been identified), become increasingly evident in tandem with IBD pathogenship, which ultimately leads to an abnormal immune response to microbial touch.

The distinction in the normal intestines between IBD and allergic reactions is a tendency to decrease inflammatory responses, such as when the intestines are inflamed in response to a potential pathogen.

As such, in people with IBD inflammation, the mucosal immune system remains permanently activated, and the intestine remains chronically inflamed.

Cytokines developed from the intestinal mucosa stimulate afferents of VN ending in the NTS (IL-1β, IL-6, TNF-α) throughout the inflammation, which transmit visceral information to activate the axis of HPA.

However, there was reported an anti-inflammatory effect of CAIP vagus efferents.

The expression of proinflammatory cytokines such as TNF-α, as stated earlier, declines at the distal end of VN efferents. Over-expression of TNF-α may be a peculiar step in IBD growth.

IBD VNS activation Vagus mitigates systemic inflammatory responses with infection of the endotoxin and intestine. The VNs also modulate the immune response of the spleen indirectly by binding to the splenic nerve.

The 3 hours of normal VNS for 5-day period for colonic rats also resulted in reduced inflammatory markers and improved signs of colitis.

Many inflammatory conditions like rheumatoid arthritis, another TNF-α-mediated disease, should also be of interest for activation of the Vagus nerve.

A study showed improvement from symptoms in patients with rheumatoid arthritis at the early and late stages of the disease by 1–4 minutes each day of VNS.

This work was also the first to show that by triggering the inflammatory reflex and increasing the frequency of symptoms, VNS inhibits the development of TNF-α and others in humans. Such evidence suggests that the vagus nerve has an anti-inflammatory role and provides people with IBDs with potential medical applications.

Positive effect of nutritional components on IBD. The role of inflammation in the production and perpetuation of psychiatric symptoms have been given mechanistic significance.

Among modern urban communities, the increase among irregular immunological responses has been associated, at least in part with, decreased exposure to commensal and environmental microorganisms that typically control immunoregulatory circuits and prevent excessive inflammation.

The bacterial intestinal flora is considered important in the growth and recurrence of IBD, and various efforts were made to modify the flora using probiotics.

Improvements have been made in animals with laboratory colitis lactobacilli treated orally or rectally.

For instance, Lactobacillus plantarum 299V prevented the onset of disease and reduced established colitis.

Furthermore, the prolibitic multi-species (VSL#3) provided normalized intestinal barrier activity to mice with proven colitis decreased proinflammatory cytokines and decreased histologic disease.

Among pets, Lactobacillus casei GG has beneficial consequences among children with moderately active CD.

In contrast, the mixture of probiotics and Saccharomyces boulardii, Lactobacillus and VSL#3 have shown a slight improvement in the effects of CD. Such results are temporary, which means that future studies need verification. No probiotic therapies have been formally approved for use with CD.

Reliable evidence is found in UC that VSL#3 is effective for mildly active pouchitis treatment. E. Coli Nissle, part of VSL#3, can be as active as a drug mesalamine in sustaining remission.

For IBD, hypnotherapy, meditation, and yoga have had a positive effect. Increasing numbers of studies have shown the advantages of relaxation-related IBD treatment.

A randomized controlled trial of a soothing workout, for instance, showed decreased pain compared to a control group and lowered anxiety level and improved quality of life.

Often useful for IBD patients were a systematic mental-body plan, mindfulness, complementary mind-body strategies, yoga, and mental-body response calming therapies.

Therefore, IBD treatment has been effective in hypnotherapy, which improves vagal tone.

Discussion A dynamic system that includes neuronal, endocrine, immune, and humoral interconnections focus on the relationship between the intestines and the brain.

The vagus nerve is unarguably an essential component of the brain-good axis that plays an important role in inflammation modulation, maintaining intestinal homeostasis, and controlling meat, satiety, and energy homeostasis consumption.

There is a well-known interaction between the food and the nerve of the vagus, and vagal tones can influence weight gain and intake.

However, in the pathogenesis of mental disorders, obesity, and other stress-induced and inflammatory diseases, the vagus nerve has an important role to play.

The vagus relaxation and several meditation techniques indicate the therapeutic effect of the vagus nerve manipulation, mainly due to its soothing and anti-inflammatory effects.

Extinction, coupled with VNS, coupled with sham stimulation, is faster than extinction. The VNS is a drug that is readily available and effective to treat severe anxiety disorders as it is already approved for insomnia and epilepsy control by the Federal FDA.

Stimulation of the vagus nerve is an effective anticonvulsant device and, in observational studies, has shown antidepressant effects for treatment resistant depression.

This mechanism can be used to interpret or exhibit multiple somatic and mental effects that describe stress-related disorders (LC, orbitocortex, insula, hippocampus, and amygdala) as the vagus nerve transmits information to areas of the brain.

Psychotropic drug products, such as serotonin reuptake inhibitors, both affect the mind and the gastrointestinal tract and should, therefore, be recognized as modulators of the brain-good axis.

Studies of nutritional absorption, somatic influences such as heart rate, physiology, and pharmacology, and vagal activity can lead to integrative treatment options like VNS, nutrition plans, medications, and behavioral therapies, such as care-giving interventions that can be adapted to individual needs.

Nerve Stimulation for Epilepsy

Treatment summary. Two forms of epilepsy stimulator systems are available. The machines in both forms transmit electrical signals to the brain to avoid the seizure-causing electrical blasts.

Under the body, below the collarbone, the vagus nerve stimulator (VNS) is inserted. Under the body, a wire (lead) connects the device to the electrodes attached to your brain's vagal nerve.

The physician is training the system to produce inadequate electrical signals that travel regularly to your brain to prevent seizures.

The reactive neurostimulator (RNS) is inserted into the skull and lead wires attach the system to the brain area that triggers the seizures.

The physician sets the system to detect unusual electrical activity in the brain and to transmit electrical signals to that brain area.

What to anticipate the stimulator of the nerve could start working immediately after the procedure. In the region where the unit is, you can find a small bulge.

And the operation will leave little scars where the wire leads have been placed and where the device has been implanted.

Why It Is Done. Nerve Stimulation could be used in some individuals who have generalized or tentative seizures, have not reacted well to antiepileptic drugs, which are not candidates for epilepsy surgery.

In combo with other treatments, nerve stimulation is used. The need for treatment is not removed by nerve stimulation. But it can help to reduce the risk of severe or frequent seizures complications.

How well it works activation of the vagus nerve decreases the occurrence of hallucinations that do not respond well to treatment and can make it less intense.

Around two out of four people say they find that after surgery they have fewer seizures. But about one out of each four people say they don't find any effects following surgery. VNS's benefits tend to increase over time.

For those who can sense when they are about to have a seizure, often turning on the VNS with their portable magnet will avoid the seizure. It may also prolong an existing seizure.

Studies show that VNS could also be effective in children. For some people whose seizures would not respond to other treatments, the responsive neurostimulator (RNS) is an option. RNS decreases seizure frequency by about half, and the effects tend to improve with time.footnote2 Risks Stimulation of the nerve is considered safe.

Many people experience side effects of the vagus nerve stimulator when the system activates the nerve. They include the following:

Coughing.

The pain of the throat.

Changes in stupidity or slight voice.

Shortness of breath.

Other possible nerve stimulator risks of both types include infection.

Tingling or numbness.

Pain, when under the skin, is the stimulator device.

What to look forward to.

Stimulation of the nerve is not a treatment for seizures, nor does it function for everyone.

The need for antiepileptic drugs is not covered by it. In an epilepsy clinic, it is most likely to be available.

HOW TO HACK YOUR VAGUS NERVE

sThe vagus nerve has a very germaine role in the body, but most men have hardly felt it. It is a long series of motor and sensory fibers extending from the brainstem to the spine, chest, and abdomen.

This nerve connects with several vital organs or processes, including the heart, lungs, intestines, liver, spleen, and kidneys.

Vagus means "moving" in Latin, appropriate for a nerve that mingles the body. It is definitely the highest in complexity of 12 pairs of cranial nerves emanating from the brain and transmits information to the tissues and organs this enters from the heart.

It's busy with the vagus nerve. There are many roles of the nervous system that are responsible for it or its related parts. Their contribution to the parasympathetic nervous system is an enormous task.

We can break the duties of the vagus nerve across four key areas: Parasympathetic–While we are at rest, this is important for body functions.

Think about things such as feeding, cycles of metabolism, and heart rate. For its function in salivation, sexual excitement, digestion, and urination, it has also been defined as the "eat and breed" or "rest and digest" process.

Sensory–It processes chest, lung, stomach, and throat sensory information.

Motor–The vagus nerve provides the neck muscles with movement that is responsible for speech and swallowing.

Special tactile–this provides a sense of tasting behind the tongue.

Of example, the vagus nerve controls multiple vital functions: maintaining a steady heart rate, coughing, sweating, controlling blood pressure and blood glucose, encouraging kidney function, pregnancy, and women's ability to reach orgasm.

It sends information to your brain about the state of your internal organs.

In fact, it deals with important functions that keep us alive.

Which occurs if the nerve of the vagus does not function well?

A little work into the vagus nerve reveals a whole host of disorders that either have been positively connected or are being examined for a correlation to the nerve.

Such vary from minor annoyances to significant issues. If you are impaired on a continuum somewhere, it can affect your overall feeling of well-being and overall performance, of course.

Many people will experience a vasovagal reaction at some point due to a vagus nerve stressor or overstimulation. Lower blood pressure, slow heart rate, and expand the legs' blood vessels, which can cause nausea or fainting.

This is a typically benign reaction, but some people who experience it more frequently may need to seek medical assistance on their own.

Other vagus-related problems include diabetes, depression, mood disorders, bradycardia, gastrointestinal diseases, chronic inflammation, fainting, and epilepsy.

Of note, most of these described factors will lead to further illness; for example, obesity and inflammation both correspond with cancers and diabetes. Disorders of anxiety or mood may also lead to depression.

How is the vagus "hacking" working?

There is a growing body of study showing that the vagus nerve can be stimulated or "hacked." Vagus hackers date back to some of Kevin Tracey's work in 1998.

In his research, he found that he could reduce the inflammatory response of the body by activating the vagus nerve with an electrical impulse.

This has positive effects on the diagnosis of illnesses like Crohn's disease, rheumatoid arthritis, and other inflammatory diseases. Research by Tracey forms the basis of the bioelectronics theory, which we now see treating disorders like anxiety and epilepsy.

Inflammation is a reaction outside of these situations that we all have in our bodies, mostly due to stress. For some people (hey, businessmen!), stress and inflammatory response may become chronic, leading to other health problems.

The vagus nerve is concerned with so many different functions that there are more "hacks" than using an external bioelectric system to activate it (usually in extreme cases only).

In fact, researchers have found that by stimulating the vagus nerve and enhancing "vagal tone," we can fight inflammation –kind of like a workout! Focus on your emotional health.

A 2010 study found that a strong vagal tone is part of a feedback loop between physical health, positive emotions, and positive social relations. With a self-sustaining system, these factors influence each other.

Participants used Loving Kindness Meditation (abbreviated as LKM) as a means to have a positive impact on their emotional health during the study. The researchers also found that it had a beneficial impact on vagal tone when people reflected on good social connections or made efforts to improve their bonds with other people.

Did you know that "good feeling" is a real thing? Vagus nerve impulses pass from the stomach to the cortex.

This has been associated with the modulation of mood and some kinds of anxiety and fear. Someone who has grace under pressure is a sign of a healthy vagal tone–a trait that most entrepreneurs could use!

The vagus nerve continuously transfers up-to-date sensory information about your body's muscles, digestive tract, heart rate, and other information across various nerves to your brain.

Research shows that our gut microbes are interlinked with those brain pathways. It is also known that gut microbiota is the immune and nervous system's possible primary modulator.

The takeaway: good health varies from person to person and depends on how you are made, but in general, you may: take probiotics, eat a healthy, balanced diet of whole foods, avoid unnecessary use of antibiotics, and minimal use of sugar or alcohol.

In fact, while probiotics are still being investigated for their effectiveness, they are shown to be an active PTSD therapy by a Canadian study.

There are also consequences of anxiety management–it can be a simple step you should do to discover whether you can benefit from taking them.

Relaxation methods penetrated Western consciousness using breathing techniques somewhere around the 1970s, but these approaches have been used by Eastern practitioners for centuries.

It points out that deep breathing is based on solid evidence–you can both relax the vagus nerve and increase the rhythm of your heart rate (HRV).

It is now widely accepted that in maintaining a healthy physiological balance, deep breathing plays a key role. "Lehrer and Gevirtz discuss a wide range of interesting theories why HRV biofeedback functions, and reaffirm that diaphragmatic breathing is definitely part of a feedback loop that increases vagal tone by activating the parasympathetic nervous system's calming response.

Notably, researchers also note that people with higher HRV (which reflects good vagal tone) had lower biomarkers for anxiety, improved psychological and physical tolerance, and stronger cognitive function. "Heavy, abdominal breathing has also been shown to suppress the" fight or flight "response during stressful situations.

Food for your vagus nerve and gut health

In addition, the vagus nerve is a pair of nerves which connects the brain with most internal organs and has a calming effect on the heart and also digestive system.

It was dubbed the superhighway between the brain and the stomach, as it easily and clearly transfers data in both directions.

Some of these stimuli influence how well you digest food and how thirsty you feel; many of them provide important information about your digestive tract's health.

The vagus nerve uses neurotransmitters called acetylcholine as messengers for relaying information along its superhighway. Therefore, for example, if the lining of the intestines involves inflammation, acetylcholine will notify the brain.

Hopefully, the brain will record that this is not an ideal long-term situation for the intestine: nutrients may not be so well absorbed, and the gut lining may become so damaged that it can no longer effectively prevent toxins from entering the bloodstream ("leaky intestine").

The vagus nerve will then transmit further acetylcholine back to the intestine with relaxing, anti-inflammatory guidance from the brain. One food for producing acetylcholine are eggs, nutritionally, it may be advisable to aid the vagus nerve function by supplying choline-containing foods so that more acetylcholine can be generated.

Egg yolks are fine choline sources if they are soft–or even better, pure, as you might see in clean, homemade mayonnaise, for example. The more egg yolks you fry, the less choline they are going to have.

Offal, like liver and kidneys, is also a good source. In either case, I would suggest a cleanliness and quality natural, pasture-fed source.

Lecithin granules (usually from soybeans, sometimes from sunflower seeds) are perfect for a vegan option to sprinkle on foods and smoothies.

Adequate consumption of L-acetyl carnitine (in food), vitamin B5 (in broccoli, chard, cabbage, sunflower seeds, and eggs) and alpha lipoic acid (in red meat, offal or brewer's yeast) can also be maintained to aid in the development of acetylcholine.

Vegetarian and those eating low amounts of meat may be able to synthesize L-acetyl carnitine from 2 amino acids: lysine as well as methionine –fish and also spirulina may be useful here.

Is the Heart Palpitations and Stomach Bloating Connected?

Can you explain that? For your heart palpitations and abdominal bloating, you saw various medical practitioners and earned a healthy health bill.

While you should be glad that you don't have a virus, you still have the issues with which you come. Your belly still bloats, and as if that were not enough, your heart starts racing as soon as it starts. Sometimes you're not lighted. What's happening?

Please note that in order to rule out serious diseases such as ovarian cancer, any unexplained stomach bloating should be reviewed by a medical professional.

How are bloating of the stomach, palpitations of the heart ,and the nerve of the vagus connected? We need to take a deeper look at the vagus nerve to know the answer.

The Irritated Vagus Nerve: How the heart, as well as stomach, are associated with cardiac palpitations have been related to digestive disorders such as IBS as well as clear cases of indigestion.

And because the vagus nerve is connected with both the digestive system and cardiac control, it is probable that excessive gas and bloating, as well as elevated cardiac activity, may be caused by, or connected.

Some have named it "vagus nerve discomfort," although it's not entirely clear which induces this collection of reactions— whether it's nerve agitation or some other warning perceived by the nerve.

Will you find that in the afternoon that you appear to bloat? Did you find that when you burp, effects subside? Is it worse in situations of stress or when you are deprived of sleep? If so, what may cause the heart to flutter may be your digestive system.

Home Remedies for Gastrointestinal Problem-Induced Heart Palpitations All of these are aimed at improving your digestive health and minimizing bloating and swelling, which will ideally also increase your heart palpitations or heart rate.

The body of everybody is different, so you might need to test out some different strategies to find the one that fits for you. Please ask your doctor to make radical changes to your diet before taking any new drugs.

Ginger capsules: For thousands of years, ginger has been used to treat digestive disorders, especially nausea stomach upset and diarrhea.

Although not well known, 550 milligrams of ginger root taken three times a day with meals that ease your bloating. If the vagus nerve itself is inflamed, ginger may be beneficial as some anti-inflammatory properties have been shown.

Burping: Any relief may be given by reducing the inflammation of the stomach. Over - the-counter goods such as

Simethicone break up gas bubbles and cause them to burp out. This is a simple short-term fix.

Switch positions: by changing your position or walking around and bending if necessary, take the pressure off your belly. If you turn about, trapped gas will escape. Experiment again. The roles that work best for you are to be sought.

Deep breathing: Depression and anxiety may be linked with nerve dysfunction of the vagus, so try to relax (I am well aware that it is easier to say than done). Try to breathe or meditate intensely.

Diet: It's a major one: it's very successful but difficult to measure. First of all, the bloating that probably caused the annoyance could be caused by a reaction to the meat.

The expulsion of the perpetrator could finally solve the problem. Gluten and milk are common gastrointestinal irritants. It can also induce gas to consume habits such as gulping the food or over-eating.

Chew your food: Chewing food thoroughly releases saliva enzymes that travel to the digestive system with the food, helping to break down the food.

Munching, which comes with inadequate enzymes, is not digested properly, leading to bloating.

Digestive enzymes: The development of enzymes reduces as you mature. If your enzyme levels are too low, the digestive process will be supplemented.

If that is the reason for the issue, it will immediately become apparent by taking an enzyme supplement.

Probiotics: Support your digestion through daily use of probiotic supplements. Using sauerkraut and kombucha, you can also replenish your gut flora with a diet rich in grown and fermented foods. If you're intolerant of lactose, try kefir.

Keep your bowels moving: taking a high-quality magnesium supplement can help if you tend to constipate. It's important to spend some money on this one and not buy in the grocery store the cheapest product.

Magnesium has many different types, and some are more bio-available than others. Here's a reference where the variations are clarified. I'm using 250 Triple Mag. Take plenty of food as well and drink plenty of water all day long.

Wishing You Good Health Researchers are still trying to understand just how our health is affected by the vagus nerve— you may encounter something that has yet to be fully understood or clarified.

Work has just started on the vagus nerve and its effects on our daily lives and the ability to use it.

That said, maybe it made you understand what's going on in your body a little bit more. Please note that a medical professional will assess any ongoing medical problem.

VAGUS NERVE DAMAGE SYMPTOMS

There are twelve cranial nerves. The vagus nerve is the longest, and some may say, the most important. The vagus nerve is vital for optimal health, no matter what the issues are.

The vagus nerve, being the longest cranial nerve, stretches from the brainstem to the stomach, going through major parts like the heart, lungs, and esophagus.

The vagus nerve contains both motor and sensory fibers and has the largest body distribution. The nerve controls involuntary processes of the body, such as regulating the heart rate and managing food.

What is the nervous illness of the vagus?

Symptoms of the vagus nerve are closely related to injury and dysfunction of the vagus nerve. You can suffer from a condition known as "gastroparesis" if your nerve is underactive.

This can lead to severe problems such as diabetes. There are several warning signs of your symptoms. This means you need to activate the vagus nerve if you experience some of the signs.

There are two types of signs of the vagus nerve. They are classified into two groups, the first being when overactive is your vagus nerve. The second group is when the nerve of your vagus is inactive or inactive.

The former group's symptoms arise as a result of the nerve's over-stimulation, while the second group's symptoms stem from little to no stimulation.

The concern is often that the signs of the vagus nerve are very close to the symptoms of IBS (irregular bowel syndrome). And it makes the diagnosis of the condition even more difficult for physicians as many of the conditions do not appear on regular testing (unless they get really bad).

But let's take a look at some of the common symptoms of vagus nerve injury so that you can recognize the disease.

The most common symptom is pain. But the pain, where it happens, and how it manifests, you really need to understand. The pain is due to a mechanical pressure, injury, or trauma that led to inflammatory swelling in your damaged vagus nerve.

The discomfort is the product of a pinched nerve in most situations (when the nerve escapes in the brain through tiny foramina). The pain you feel is flat and ambiguous, not like someone is poking you relentlessly and painfully.

Dysfunction of the organs, as stated at the outset, the vagus nerve is the longest cranial nerve, flowing through several vital organs. These organs can't receive the signals and information that your body sends when the nerve is damaged.

You will notice localized symptoms of organ dysfunction due to damage to nerve fibers. That doesn't mean your organs are going to suddenly stop working, but some of them are going to work less.

Muscle cramps

One of the vagus nerve's main functions is to provide the vocal cord muscles with sensation. Some trauma or vagus nerve dysfunction will also cause damage to these muscles. The injury affects the voice and breathing.

It will also affect any other organs that are assisted by the vagus nerve. Although you may assume that the cause of your muscle cramps is a low amount of electrolytes (such as magnesium as well as potassium), it might be that the cause is damage to your vagus nerve.

Swallowing difficulties As described above, the nerve of the vagus starts at the brainstem and travels through your whole body. The nerve causes the expression of your cough.

People with trauma to the vagus nerve experience difficulty swallowing just as patients suffering from a head injury or stroke have trouble swallowing. You may find an imbalance in your gag reflex, and that may cause you to panic when feeding. The general difficulty of swallowing is only the beginning.

Fainting

One of the most serious symptoms of the vagus nerve is fainting, which happens when the brain becomes overactive and over-stimulated. You are having sudden fainting and fall events. Although it is not life-threatening to faint on its own, fainting increases the risk of accidental injury.

Peptic ulcer

Another disease that may occur as a result of injury to the vagus nerve is peptic ulcer. The damage may affect the normal mechanisms of control that are responsible for the secretion of gastric acid.

As a consequence, you can undergo prolonged peptic acid secretion, leading to ulceration and other gastro-related diseases and conditions (e.g., dyspepsia and gastroesophageal reflux disease).

I stated this disorder earlier in Gastroparesis. And we're going to end the list of symptoms of the vagus nerve. This disease arises because of the nerve's inactivity. The result is blood supply interference to the stomach after food ingestion.

Simply put, you're suffering from poor digestion. The symptoms that you will feel are painful abdominal spasms that may cause weight loss, nausea, and heartburn, affecting your normal intake of food.

Treating vagus nerve problems

I advise that you start treating the condition once you begin to experience any of the symptoms. Many of the therapies also help prevent injury to the vagus nerve.

The first and most common therapy is the stimulation of the vagus nerve.

When the injury is serious, at least in terms of operation, you need to activate the vagus nerve with a system that is very close to the cardiac pacemaker.

This system is inserted under your body. But even before the disorder becomes serious, you can stimulate your vagus nerve.

Vagus nerve stimulation has shown positive outcomes for problems such as anxiety disorders, heart disease, Adhd, migraines, diabetes, bulimia, memory disturbances, severe heart failure, mood disorders, leaky bowel, impaired blood circulation, Alzheimer's and more.

So the question now is: how can you activate the nerve of the vagus? Options include a cold shower, singing or chanting, meditation, yoga, positive social relationships, laughter, breathing exercises, fasting, massage, deep and slow breathing, tai chi, sleeping on your right side, praying, chewing gum, acupuncture, and tensioning your stomach muscles.

Medical experts consider using a feeding tube in the case of severe gastroparesis to deliver food directly to the intestines to avoid malnutrition.

Several drugs are also being used. Of example, of fainting, medical experts advise using medications to treat the symptoms of fainting. Sertraline and paroxetine are some of the popular options.

Reflex syncope

Because of a neurologically mediated drop in blood pressure, involuntary syncope is a temporary loss of consciousness. There may be sweating, a decreased vision to see, or ringing in the ears before the person goes out.

Occasionally, if subconscious, the person can twitch. Complications may include fall injuries.

There are three forms of reflex syncope: vasovagal, acute, and carotid sinus. Usually, vasovagal syncope is caused by seeing blood, suffering, emotional stress, or prolonged standing. Usually, urination, swallowing, or coughing triggers situational syncope.

The syncope of the carotid sinus is due to pressure in the neck on the carotid sinus.

The underlying mechanism entails slowing the heart rate by the nervous system and dilating blood vessels resulting in low blood pressure and thus not enough blood flow to the brain. Upon leaving out other possible causes, treatment is based on symptoms.

Without specific treatment, recovery occurs. Prevention is to stop the stimuli. It may also be beneficial to drink adequate water, salt, and exercise.

If this is not appropriate for vasovagal syncope, it is possible to try drugs such as midodrine or fludrocortisone. A heart pacemaker may be used from time to time.

Reflex syncope affects at least one person every 1,000 a year. It is the commonest type of syncope, representing more than 50% of all cases.

Signs and symptoms

Vasovagal syncope episodes are normally chronic and usually occur when exposed to a particular stimulus by the predisposed patient.

Until losing consciousness, the patient frequently exhibits early signs or symptoms such as lightheadedness, vomiting, feeling extremely hot or cold (accompanied with sweating), ringing in the ears, an unpleasant sensation in the chest, confused feelings, agitation, a mild inability to speak or form sentences (sometimes associated with noticeable stuttering), fatigue and visual disruption.

Over several seconds to a number of minutes before the loss of consciousness, the effects may become more severe. It normally happens when a person is standing or sitting up.

When people lose their consciousness, they hit the floor (unless prevented) and, in this position, immediately restore effective blood flow to the brain, allowing the person to regain consciousness.

If the patient does not collapse into a completely flat, supine position, and the head remains raised above the spine, a seizure-like syndrome can result from the failure of the blood to return to the brain rapidly, and the body's nerves may shoot off and generally cause muscles to twitch quite slightly, but mostly stay very rigid.

The physical status of the autonomic nervous system (see below) leading to a loss of consciousness can continue for several minutes, so if people try to sit or stand up as they wake up, they will vanish again.

The person may be nauseated, weak, and sweating for several minutes or hours. The subsequent loss of blood to the brain causes fainting as heart rate increases, or blood pressure decreases.

Vasovagal syncope Common stimuli includes:

- Long-standing
- Emotional Pressure
- Pain
- Blood vision
- Time changing magnetic field (i.e., transcranial magnetic stimulation)
- Situational syncope After or during urination (micturition syncope) straining, such as bowel movement
- Coughing
- Lifting a heavy weigh
- Carotid sinus syncope
- Pressing at some point in the chest. This can happen if you wear a close tie, shave, or turn your head.

Pathophysiology Whatever the cause, the syncope process is identical in the different syndromes of the vasovagal syncope.

The nucleus tractus solitarii of brainstem is manipulated directly or indirectly by the initiating signal, resulting in parasympathetic nervous system (vagal) tone change concurrently and loss of sympathetic nervous system sound.

This results in a continuum of hemodynamic responses: cardioinhibitory reaction at one end of the spectrum is characterized by a reduction in heart rate (negative chronotropic effect) and contractility (negative inotropic effect) contributing to a decline in cardiac output that is sufficiently important to contribute to a loss of consciousness.

This response is thought to be primarily the result of improving the parasympathetic tone.

On the second end of the spectrum is the response of the vasodepressor, caused by a drop in blood pressure (up to 80/20) without much heart rate change.

It phenomenon occurs due to blood vessel dilation, probably due to the loss of the sympathetic tone of the nervous system.

Somewhere between these two ends of the spectrum, many individuals with vasovagal syncope have a mixed response.

The Bezold-Jarisch reaction is one reason for these physiological responses.

Vasovagal syncope can be a response to evolution, specifically the response to fight or flight.

Diagnosis A variety of other medical conditions may induce syncope, in addition to the process mentioned above.

It is hard to make the right diagnosis for the loss of consciousness. The core of vasovagal syncope diagnosis is based on a clear description of a typical pattern of triggers, symptoms, and timing.

Differentiating lightheadedness, nausea, vertigo, and low blood sugar as other factors are important.

Diagnostic accuracy can often be improved in people with recurrent vasovagal syncope by one of the following diagnostic tests;

A tilt test (results should be interpreted in the context of clinical presentations of patients and with a comprehension of the sensitivity and specificity of the test) Implantation of an insertable loop recorder. A Holter monitor or even an event monitor (an echocardiogram.)

Changes in lifestyle

The foundation of recovery is to eliminate stimuli in that person known to cause syncope. Nevertheless, studies have shown that, if the cause is psychological or cognitive, e.g., blood vision, people show significant decreases in vasovagal syncope by exposure-based interventions with counselors.

However, if the trigger is a particular drug, then the only treatment is avoidance.

In those who have syncope with blood flow, a technique known as "applied pressure" may also be helpful.

The technique is performed by tightening the skeletal muscles when the exposure occurs for about 15 seconds and then slowing them down. This is done for a few minutes every 30 seconds.

Since vasovagal syncope allows blood pressure to drop, it is not advisable to relax the whole body as a method of avoidance.

A patient should raise or cross the legs and relax the muscles of the legs so that blood pressure does not fall too dramatically before an injection.

The affected person may increase the intake of salt and fluids to increase the volume of blood before established triggering events. It may be good to have sports drinks or electrolyte drinks.

People ought to be enlightened on how to respond to additional syncope events, particularly if they encounter symptoms of prodromal warning: they should lie down and lift their arms, or at least lower their heads to improve blood flow to the brain.

At the very least, the patient should try to relocate to a 'safe,' possibly cushioned, location in case of loss of consciousness, upon the onset of initial symptoms. It is ideal to position yourself in a way that minimizes the impact of falling or collapsing. The 'healthy' place should be near, because time is of concern, and these symptoms usually occur in a matter of minutes to lose consciousness.

If the patient has lost consciousness, his or her head turned to the side should be laid down. It is important to undo tight clothing. If the trigger element is known, it should be omitted (for example, the source of pain) once possible.

It can be advantageous to wear graded compression stockings.

Medicines Some medicines may also be helpful: beta blockers (β-adrenergic antagonists) were once the most common medicines given; however, they have been shown to be ineffective in a variety of studies and are therefore no longer prescribed.

However, by reducing blood pressure and heart rate, they can induce syncope.

Medicines that may be active include: fludrocortisone, midodrine, CNS stimulants, SSRIs such as paroxetine or sertraline, disopyramide, and atropine epinephrine (adrenaline) in health care environments where a syncope is expected.

The implantation of a permanent pacemaker can be positive or even curative for patients with the cardioinhibitory form of vasovagal syncope.

Long-term vasovagal syncope treatment types include.

Preloading agents; Vasoconstrictors Anticholinergic agents negative cardiac inotropes Central agents Mechanical device Discontinuation of drugs known to lower blood pressure might be helpful, but in some people stopping antihypertensive drugs may also be dangerous.

Using antihypertensive medications may make the syncope worse as the depression may have been the way the body can pay back for the low blood pressure.

Prognosis

Normally, short periods of unconsciousness do not cause any lasting harm to health. Even in very healthy individuals, reflex syncope can happen and has several possible causes, mostly insignificant ones such as extended standing.

The main risk of vasovagal syncope (or vertigo dizzy spells) is the risk of injury from falling unconscious.

Medication treatment may prevent future vasovagal reactions; however, medication is unsuccessful for some individuals, and they will continue to experience fainting episodes.

THE VAGUS NERVE IN TRAUMA RECOVERY

The body feels other distressing signs of post-traumatic stress— a tightness in the chest, a deep sensation in the abdomen, a comfortable pain in the mouth, or a constant sense of fatigue.

They now understand that as part of the healing process, they will turn to the body, and as a result, we have seen a rise in the use of meditation, mindfulness, tai chi, Qigong, Feldinkreis, massage, craniosacral therapy, and acupuncture in post-traumatic stress disorder.

Such mind-body treatments are helping us to be less passive, less sensitive, and less impulsive to pain. We are raising our consciousness of the options we need to make us feel grounded and peaceful.

We feel in control more. Stimulating the vagus nerve is a method that mind-body treatments operate. Knowledge of how this nerve functions offers a basic understanding of traumatic stress and promotes our healing capacity.

As a consequence, the vagus nerve has become central to the diagnosis for trauma.

The use of mind-body therapy was associated with a wide range of enhancements in well-being including:

Gains in physical and mental health. Increased opiate and psychotropic use. Enhanced psychological well-being.

Better social interactions. Reduced autonomic sympathetic function. Reduced blood pressure. Improved neuroendocrine activity. Improved thyroid health. Improved blood sugar control.

Several mechanisms help explain how symptoms relieve mind-body therapies. We allow us to focus on our emotional feelings, desires, and motives.

This observational capacity helps to increase awareness of discomfort and may result in reduced emotional reactivity, fear, nausea, chronic pain, and depression. In contrast, mental-body interventions improve self-compassion and the capacity to compassionately perceive the point of view of another person.

Therefore, mental-body treatments are successful as they include physiological changes in the adaptive nervous system as determined by changes in the vagus nerve structure.

The vagus nerve passes through the muscles of the head, inner ear, throat, chest, lungs, abdomen, and intestines from the brainstem. Mind-body therapies produce changes with how we orient ourselves towards our environment by bringing a soft gaze and inviting us to explore new breath or movement patterns that interact directly with these body areas.

One way researchers calculate the changes that occur in the vagus nerve is also referred to as respiratory sinus arrhythmia by heart rate variability (HRV).

HRV refers to your heart rate's rhythmic oscillations that arise with your breath.

It is a function of your heartbeat cycles. Increased variation in heart rate is associated with increased ability to tolerate or rebound from stress, while lower variance in heart rate is correlated with stress and anxiety.

You should think of any form of mind-body therapy that enhances the variation in heart rate as creating mobility and endurance within the autonomic nervous system.

As a result, switching between feelings of anticipation and relaxation is smoother.

Trauma and the vagus nerve

They change the way they breathe when we face a risk (real or perceived). Here, by thinking about how animals react to predators, we can get a clear picture.

In some situations, an individual may immediately breathe into the upper chest, a calming reaction to the nervous system that helps them to run or fight in a threatening situation.

In other situations, an individual may stop in order to avoid being detected by a predator, which means breathing shallowly or holding breath.

The freeze reflex allows the individual to stand still, which is a response to the threat of immobilization. In some situations, animals may become vulnerable so that a predator who is not a scavenger can lose interest in a dead animal.

An evolutionarily older pathway of both the vagus nerve as well as part of the parasympathetic nervous system facilitates both the freezing and faint responses.

More significantly, when healthy, by shaking and breathing in a manner that maintains homeostasis, an individual can trigger the stress response.

Nevertheless, for extended periods of time, we humans will often linger in both high activation (fight and flight) and low activation (freeze and faint) responses.

It tends to be the case where trauma is persistent and recurrent, as in the case of Complex PTSD. However, there are often inadequate resources for handling painful or upsetting experiences. This can result in physical stress and restricted breathing patterns that form the basis for our posture, modes of motion, and general self-sense.

The Vagus Nerve and Trauma Recovery

A three-part hierarchical structure includes the autonomic nervous system: the dorsal vagal system, the sympathetic nervous system, and the ventral vagal system.

When part of the parasympathetic nervous system, the dorsal vagal system, which is the youngest of the processes. By encouraging a shutdown reflex, the dorsal vagal nerve immobilizes the body in response to life-threatening situations.

By activating the fight-or-flight response, the sympathetic nervous system, which is comparatively newer to evolve, mobilizes the body to respond to threats.

Perhaps specifically, mental-body interventions help activate the ventral vagal system, which is the systems' newest and most advanced.

This system of "social engagement" is the branch of the parasympathetic nervous system that helps you relax when you feel safe and connect with others.

To enable reset your vagus nerve, you can learn practices; however, it's not like every practice is correct for everyone. Instead, I encourage you to test and start exploring a variety of practices in breathing and movement until you find out what works for you.

You will start learning techniques through a process of self-study and conscious body awareness that helps you maintain a sense of security and recover from trauma.

Here are some resources to help you get started: Visit your Gut: By maintaining a healthy digestive system, you can also improve the protection of your vagus nerve.

The internal nervous system, also known as the belly brain, consists of the "microbiome" in your stomach.

This habitat includes hundreds of good and bacterial organisms living within the intestinal tracts.

A deficiency in your intestine will result in an inflammatory response in your immune system, causing a wide range of debilitating effects, including anxiety and depression.

Through increasing the intake of sugar and finding any latent food intolerances, you will create a healthy microbiota.

You may need a physician or nutritionist's help in identifying the causes of an intestinal deficiency, but the time it takes to incorporate these improvements into your life is well worth it.

Laughing Aloud. It has been said that "laughter is the best medicine". It creates a natural rush in endorphins all over the skin. A good laugh on the belly automatically affects your breathing, heart rate, and blood pressure.

Laughter is an activity based on the body; it produces facial, chest, diaphragm, and belly movement. Keep on the lookout for a diversion of music, a friendly mate, or a decent comedian to give a good workout to your vagus nerve.

Shake it Out. Inspired by wild animals, you can use a quick method of shaking to let go of emotional stress or get out of a freeze reaction.

Next, check your body to find points of stress with your consciousness. So concentrate on these spots and encourage yourself to shake them out one at a time.

Let yourself yield to the trembling and emit any sounds that accompany the action if necessary. Take a moment to stop in silence when you feel complete and note the resulting release.

The nerve of the Honeybee Breath Vagus passes through vocal and inner ear chords. Humming and singing can therefore have a calming effect on your nervous system. Throughout yoga, the breath of Bhamari pranayama, or Honeybee, is an opportunity to experiment with a buzzing rhythm.

In this lesson, I encourage you to pose with your palms (thumbs facing down) in a comfortable position and close your ears. Build a humming sound on the exhale to vibrate your eardrum. Repeat as long as you want.

Rinse and Repeat In reality, the vagus nerve continually pushes us into and out of equilibrium as we always respond to our world's shifting demands.

Hence, we often have to repeat exercises of vagus nerve balancing. That is why as a daily practice, most mind-body treatments are used.

In fact, we need to be safe and feel safe to be effective with these activities. Occasionally our body's signals warn us we're not healthy.

In this case, to protect ourselves, we need to honor the message that often requires us to make changes in our lives.

Through comparison, there may be occasions when we respond in the form of flashbacks to experiences of traumatic trauma.

In this case, in order to heal from past wounds, it may be necessary to work with a therapist who specializes in trauma treatment. Alternatively, the vagus nerve's "imbalances" are likely to return until the root issues are addressed and fixed.

CONCLUSION

All deductions written in this book were from real scientific research done in the past. All advice, precautions, and notes should be put to practice as per stated procedures. In special cases, please see your Doctor.

www.ingramcontent.com/pod-product-compliance
Lightning Source LLC
Chambersburg PA
CBHW060834220526
45466CB00003B/1095